THE COMPLETE MAKEUP AND BEAUTY BOOK

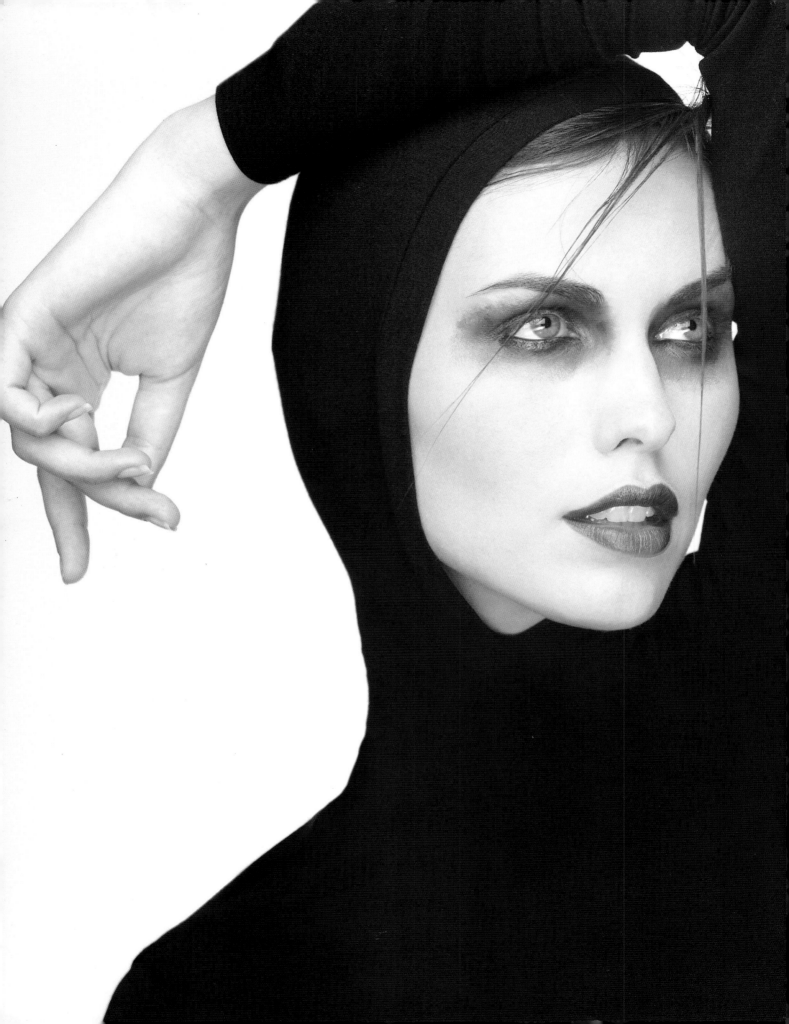

THE COMPLETE MAKEUP AND BEAUTY BOOK

LEIGH TOSELLI

Photography by Patrick Toselli

First published in 2004 by New Holland Publishers
London ● Cape Town ● Sydney ● Auckland
www.newhollandpublishers.com

86 Edgware Road
London, W2 2EA
United Kingdom

14 Aquatic Drive
Frenchs Forest
NSW 2086, Australia

80 McKenzie Street
Cape Town, 8001
South Africa

218 Lake Road
Northcote, Auckland
New Zealand

ISBN 1 84330 878 9

Although the publishers have made every effort to ensure that the information
contained in this book was correct at the time of going to press, they accept
no responsibility for any inaccuracies, loss, injury or inconvenience sustained
by any person using this book as reference.

Publishing managers: Claudia dos Santos, Simon Pooley
Commissioning editors: Alfred LeMaitre, Ingrid Corbett
Publisher: Mariëlle Renssen
Editor: Sandra Cattich
Concept and design: Petal Palmer
Beauty consultant: Beryl Barnard
Production: Myrna Collins

Reproduction by Hirt & Carter (Pty) Ltd
Printed and bound in Singapore by Tien Wah Press (Pte) Limited

10 9 8 7 6 5 4 3 2 1

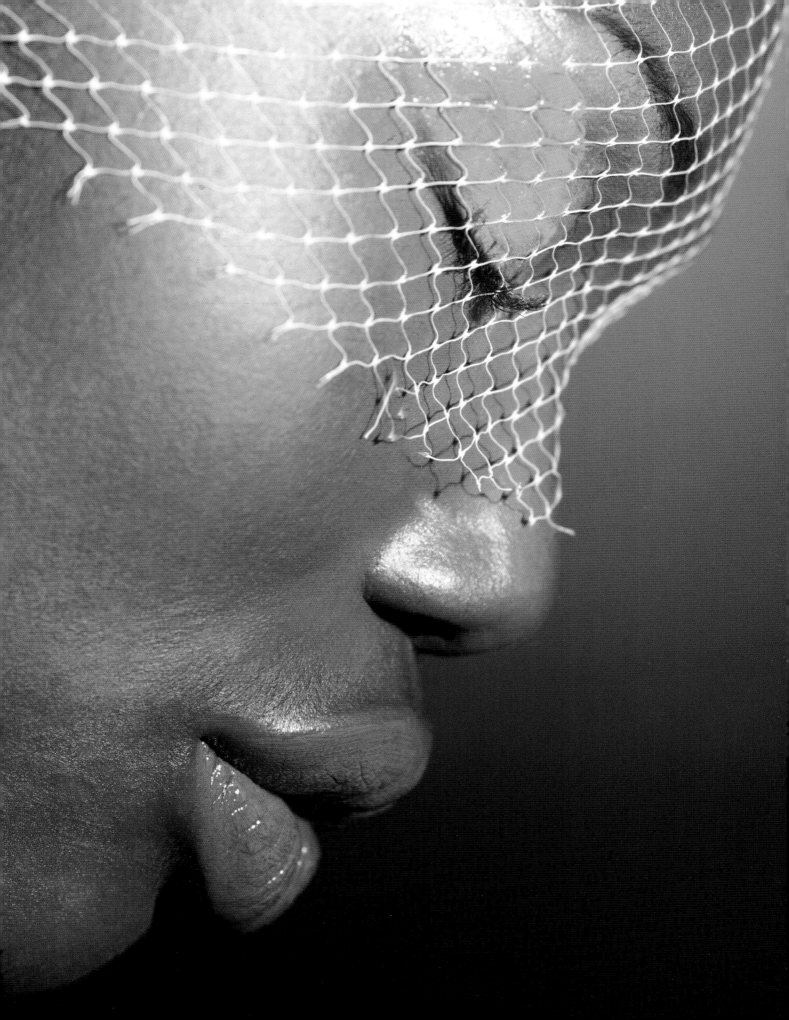

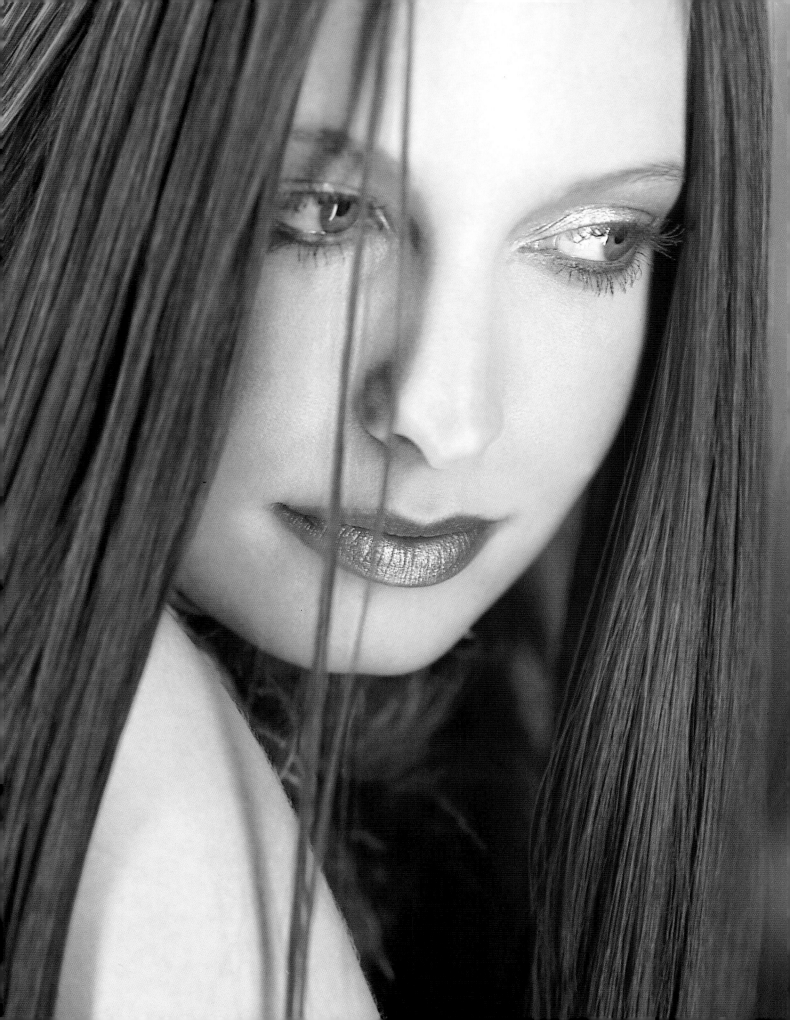

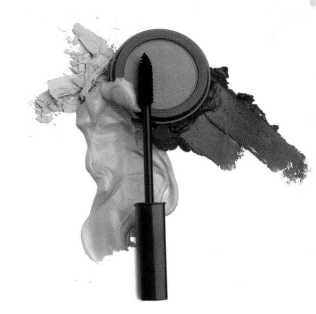

CONTENTS

INTRODUCTION

Catwalk and fashion editorials are meant to inspire and innovate, but very often fashion statements can be taken to extremes – from following whatever the magazines portray, to holding onto looks that are long out of date. Finding a balance between fashion, comfort and personal style is the most logical solution.

Thibault Vabre, an international make-up artist for Clarins, maintains, "If a woman's make-up is successful, you don't see it, you see the person". Learn to make the most of your features and find out what make-up looks compliment you – after all, big noses, full lips, gappy teeth and moles have all been turned into beauty trademarks over the years. Decide what suits you – you are the expert! So whether you've never worn make-up at all, whether you are pretty adept at doing your own face or whether you are stuck in a rut, this book will help alleviate any nervousness you might have about make-up application and will provide you with lots of inspiration, tips and ideas to help you attain exciting new looks.

Instead of looking in a mirror and asking "What's wrong with me?", use make-up to highlight your uniqueness, not to hide and correct. Just remember to keep it simple – when you try too hard it looks complicated and unnatural. Find your own basic make-up essentials to create a radiant-looking complexion, and experiment with different products and tools to accentuate your best features. Improving your appearance will boost your confidence and self-esteem. Ultimately, it's not about what rules to follow, but about learning how to adapt the various techniques to best suit your own unique style. Experimentation is fun, and besides, you can always wash it off!

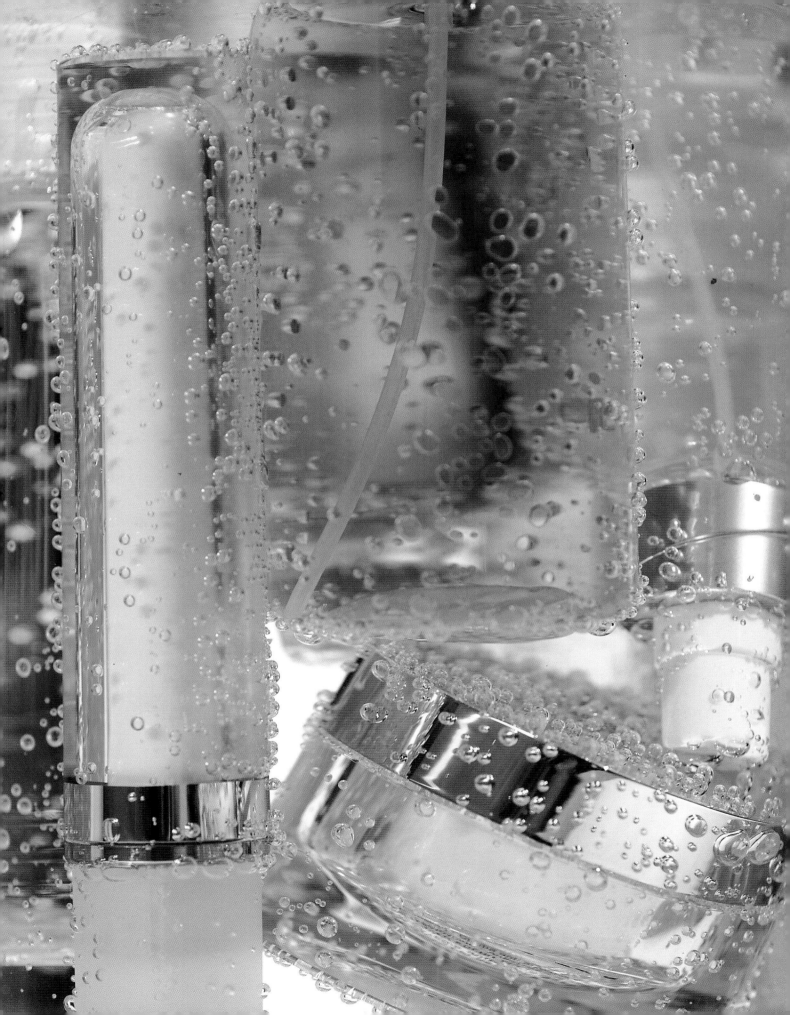

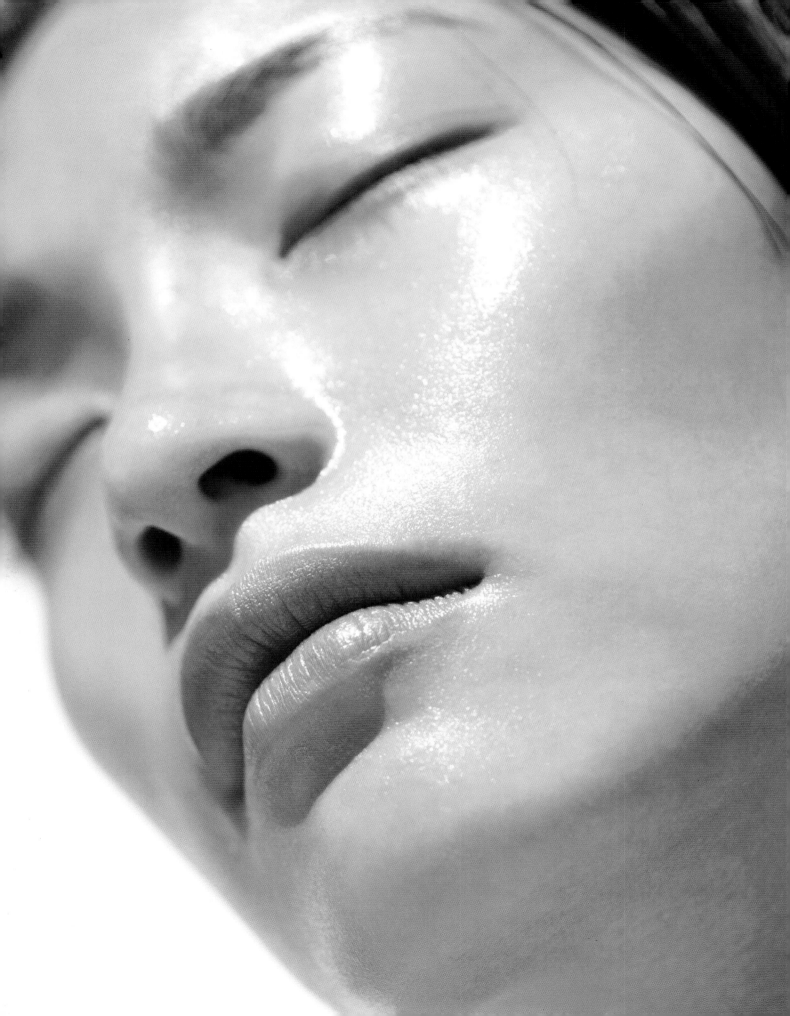

part one

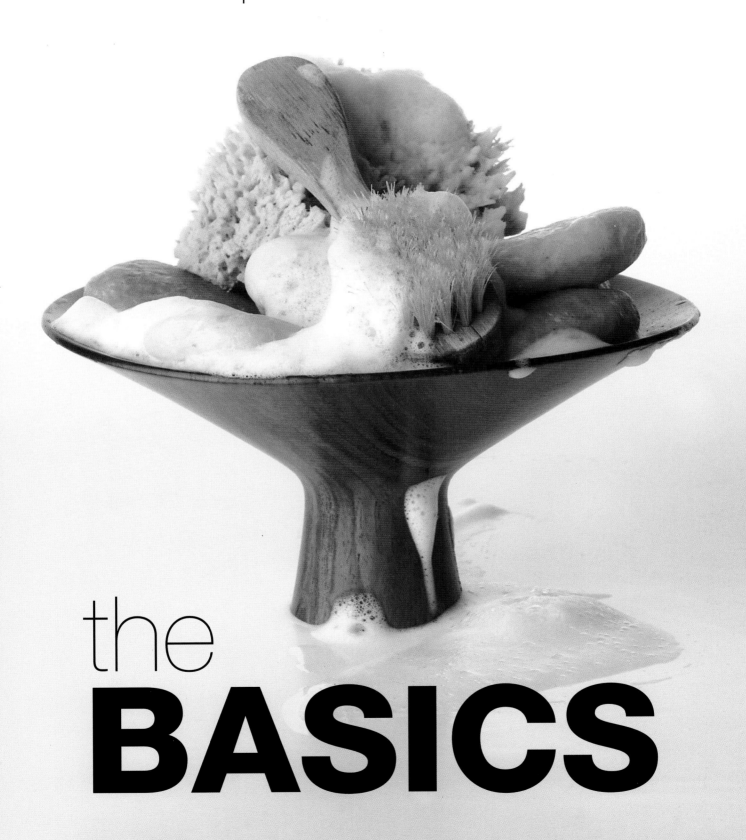

the
BASICS

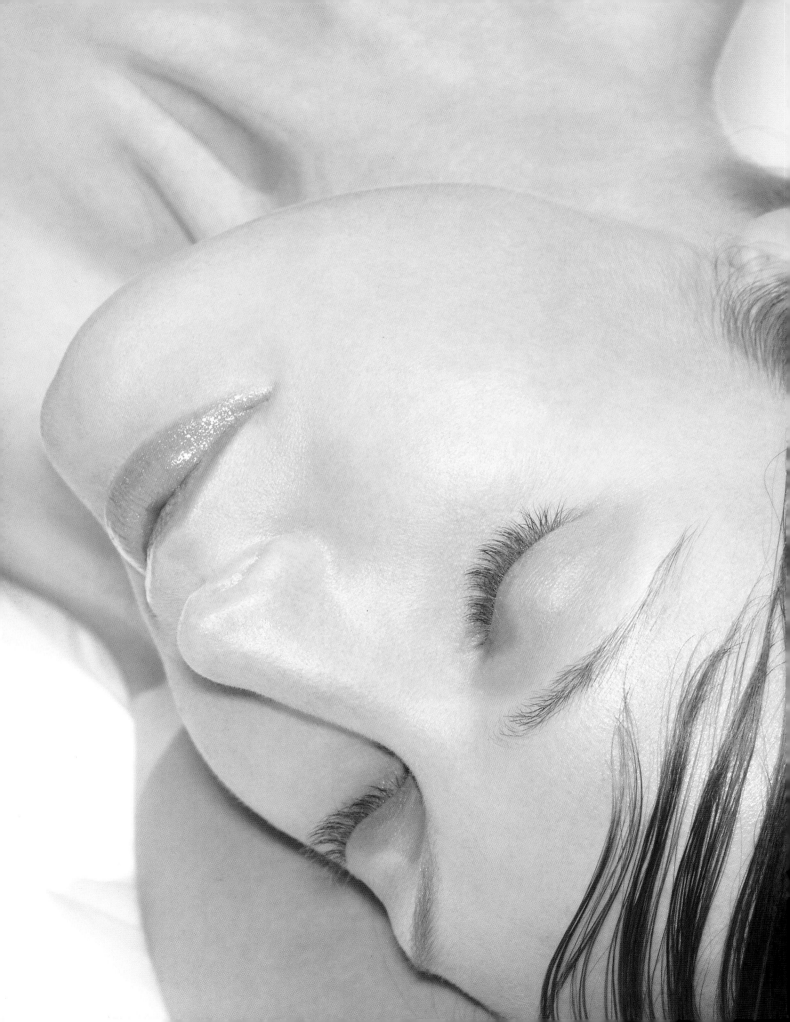

As humans, you come packaged in material that's light, tough, elastic and waterproof. Your skin protects your body against the world. It also plays a large part in how people respond to you. Depending on the state of your skin, you may be met with snap judgements on your health and sexual attractiveness. So it's no wonder that a multimillion-dollar industry has grown up around skin sensitivities.

Weighing about 4kg (6.6lb), the skin is the largest organ in the body. It covers roughly 2m^2 (6.6 sq ft) and consists of 3 layers. Like no other material, it grows with you, repairs itself and processes sensory information about the environment. It acts as a barrier against pollution, radiation, the elements, harmful micro-organisms and physical trauma.

Smooth, poreless and free from lines, a flawless complexion has long been considered a mark of youthfulness and good looks. No part of our body receives as much attention as our skin; we slather it with creams, conceal it with make-up, and examine every change, line and blemish.

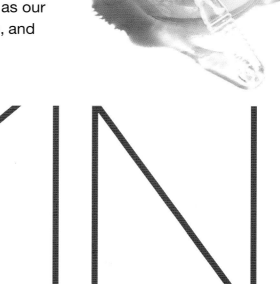

SKIN

" For some, achieving perfect skin seems impossible, but good skin is achievable. It simply takes work! With a bit of knowledge, your skin will look better – and be healthier – than you ever thought possible ... "

YOUR SKIN TYPE

The term 'skin type' refers to two things: how much sebum your skin produces, and where this sebum is most heavily produced. But our skin changes – greasy one day and dry the next. It's under constant attack from internal factors like fluctuating hormones and poor diet, which lead to oiliness and spots, and from external factors like the sun and the wind, which cause premature wrinkles.

Factors such as stress and the changing seasons can also take their toll, making skin look dull, flaky and lifeless. To combat these enemies, skin needs to be properly cared for throughout your life. Examine your skin first thing in the morning to identify your skin type and discover which products to use and which to avoid.

Dry skin

Avoid
- sun exposure, which aggravates the condition; excessive lubrication; and products containing alcohol and fragrance.

Look for
- products containing sealants to prevent moisture loss such as silicone or collagen; daytime protective moisturizers; nourishing and hydrating masks; products containing vitamin E, avocado oil, hyaluronic acid and ceramides.

Oily skin

Avoid
- harsh strippers with a high alcohol content; foundations with a 'glossy' or 'satin finish'; harsh alcohol-based toners; soap and water; oil-based moisturizers; and finally, touching your face too much.

Look for
- 'oil-free' foundations and moisturizers; products labelled non-comedogenic and non-acnegenic; antibacterial essential oils such as tea tree and grapefruit; and cleansing oils, rather than rich creams and lotions.

Dry skin

Most people try to combat dry skin by saturating it with oil – not the best plan when you realize that dry skin is actually thirsty skin. What you need is a regular supply of water – at least eight glasses of water a day – and creams that contain water.

Air conditioning and wind exposure aggravate dry skin, so apply moisturizer at least twice a day, and give yourself the occasional intensive night treatment.

Dry skin doesn't retain moisture well as it produces few protective oils – no visible surface oil. Dehydrated skin is different – it's a symptom of an overall drought in your system. Signs include ultra-fine crisscross lines over the cheek areas and the presence of oily areas.

Oily skin

An oily skin has definite advantages; it's a natural moisturizer that protects the epidermis from in- and outdoor climates so that you won't age quickly. But excess sebum has its downfalls too. It leaves the skin prone to seborrhoea (too much oil), which brings open pores and break-outs.

People with oily skin tend to overwash and overstimulate the skin, which only serves to increase the activity of the sebaceous glands, resulting in more sebum production.

Combination skin

All skin is essentially combination skin. It is usually plump and evenly coloured, but may have a slight oily panel across the nose, chin and forehead, or T-zone. Quite a few of us have large pores and lots of oil around the nose, chin, and perhaps the forehead. But we also have normal or dry skin under the eyes and on the cheeks. To treat combination skin, you treat the two zones separately, giving the oily bits the sebum-absorbing care they need, and moisturizing the dry or normal bits.

Combination skin

Avoid

- harsh products for the T-zone; exfoliating scrubs; leaving make-up on overnight; and strong-alcohol-based toners.

Look for

- nourishing masks as treats; night cream to maximize beauty sleep, and moisturizers with sun protection.

Sensitive skin

While sensitive skin is a skin condition rather than a skin type, it is true that some skin – regardless of whether it is oily, dry or combination – is easily irritated and shows red, dry patches where the skin has started to flake.

Sensitive skin

Avoid

- products containing alcohol; surfactants (detergents used in certain cleansers and soaps); fragrances and some plant extracts. Stay out of the sun and protect yourself with high-factor sunscreens.

Look for

- products labelled hypoallergenic or containing skin soothers such as kaolin, camomile and aloe.

What's your skin type?

When you know your skin type, you'll be able to buy the right cleanser, exfoliator and moisturizer.

1. After washing my skin feels:
  a. so tight that it hurts to smile
  b. clean, but it gets shiny 20 minutes later
  c. just fine
  d. slightly shiny 20 minutes later, only on the T-zone

2. When I don't use a night cream, my skin looks:
  a. rough and flaky
  b. rather oily
  c. same as it did the night before
  d. slightly shiny only on the T-zone

3. The pores on my T-zone are:
  a. nearly invisible, even when I look in the mirror
  b. clearly visible when I stand 30cm (11.7in) from the mirror
  c. only visible close up or with a magnifying mirror
  d. somewhat visible in a regular mirror

Mostly **a** answers = dry skin
Mostly **b** answers = oily skin
Mostly **c** answers = normal skin
Mostly **d** answers = combination skin

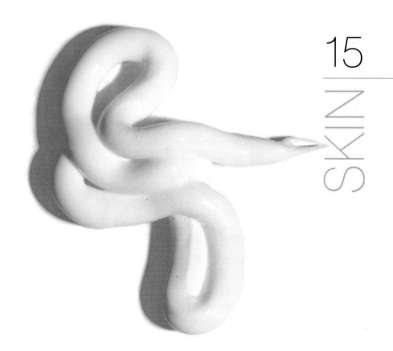

SKIN-CARE NECESSITIES

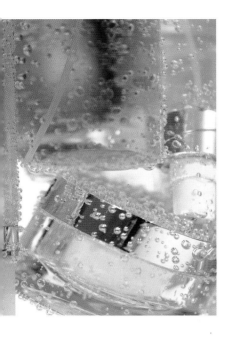

Skin-care technology has grown in leaps and bounds, allowing us to manipulate our skins in ways never before possible. Today mattifying agents can improve oily skin, retinoids can erase the years and full-spectrum sunscreens mean protection all year round.

Yet increased awareness and the proliferation of beauty products has led to a lot of confusion when it comes to skin care. Bathroom cabinets are filled to capacity with every imaginable cream and improver, yet problems persist.

Perhaps it's time to get back to basics, to really listen to your skin. Making the effort to understand the effects that lifestyle, stress, the environment and time can have on the appearance of your skin is crucial. Only then can you make informed choices and start to reap the benefits.

As you know by now, there is no good make-up without good skin. Make-up should enhance your natural beauty, not mask it. Taking responsibility for your skin, means getting into a proper regime and looking after it correctly each and every day.

The better you take care of yourself and your skin, the better you look. Although you can't change your genetic make-up, you can be kind to your body (sleep, water and healthy food) and you can control your skin's condition.

SLEEP
Try going without it and you'll see why you need it so desperately. Under-eye circles and bags are just the beginning.

WATER
Whether it's drinking eight glasses a day, washing twice a day or hydrating whenever you need it – water is crucial.

SUNSCREEN
To avoid wrinkles, sunburn, brown spots, cancer protect your face with one of the new foundations containing built-in sun protection. Even a basic foundation creates some protection from the sun's rays.

DON'T SMOKE
Never mind what it's doing to your lungs, smoking causes wrinkles, especially around the mouth.

TAKE IT OFF
Leaving make-up on overnight clogs pores and is probably the worst thing you can do to your skin.

HEALTHY FOOD
Avoid processed food, which is full of chemicals and preservatives.

Eat a diet rich in antioxidant nutrients: you will find vitamins A, C and E in dairy products, citrus fruits, green vegetables and vegetable oil.

The minerals selenium, zinc and magnesium in fish, nuts, pulses, milk, poultry and wholemeal breads, help combat free radicals.

MOISTURE
Whether you opt for a gel, a cream or a lotion, you will need a moisturizer that suits your skin type. Anything too rich or unsuitable will simply block pores and create unsightly problems.

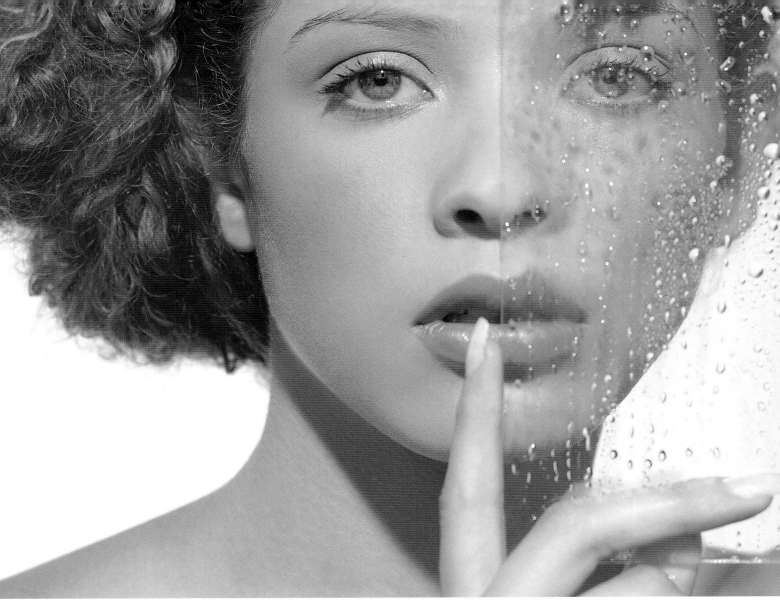

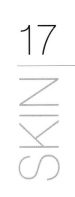

"Sleep and water are essential to great looking skin."

SKIN CARE

A clear, glowing, healthy complexion is an ideal that we all aspire to. Some are luckier than others, but whether you're trying to improve the skin you've got or just maintain it, understanding how your skin functions, and what is actually happening when it starts to wrinkle or develop spots, will definitely help.

Your skin is a protective barrier against harmful external substances such as bacteria, chemicals and UV (ultraviolet) rays. It also helps to retain electrolytes (minerals lost in perspiration) and other essential body fluids. Whatever your particular skin type, there are three basic factors you need to bear in mind if you want a youthful-looking skin. You will need to cleanse regularly, hydrate properly and protect your skin from the elements before you address any of the problems that relate to your particular skin type.

Cleansing

If you want your skin to look and feel great, careful cleansing is important; after all, cleanliness is next to godliness, or so say ancient scriptures and over-zealous parents. True, nothing beats that freshly washed feeling, but there's a fine line between a clean complexion and a scrubbed one. The latter does little to raise your beauty profile and plenty to destroy your skin's pH balance.

Choosing the right cleanser can be daunting. There are wash-off gels, AHA (alpha-hydroxy acid) rinse-way liquid gels, tissue-off cleansing milks, and soap-free bars. If you experience spots, dry or sensitive skin, it's worth looking very closely at your cleansing regime. Too much cleansing can cause problems with the protective layers if you are constantly stripping away essential oils.

Soap can dry the skin because it dissolves and washes away skin oils or lipids that seal the skin's dead, horny layer. Normal skin should be able to make up this lipid deficiency within a few hours, but dry skin often can't generate enough lipids to make up the shortfall before you next wash your face.

Skin is naturally acidic with a pH balance of around 5.5, soap is generally alkaline with a pH of 8 or higher. If you use soap with hard water you will find it difficult to rinse off. The residue left behind can upset the skin's natural acid balance and may continue to dry out skin lipids long after the washing process is over.

Cosmetic cleansers are formulated to dissolve the most stubborn of make-up formulations, excess skin oils and dirt. The best cleanser is one that leaves skin lipids in place so that your skin feels supple and fresh without any clogged pores. In the past cleansing milks and lotions were prescribed for dry skins, while foaming washes or non-soap bars were indicated for oilier skins, but with the numerous choices available, texture and preferences are really up to you.

I'd suggest using formulations that rinse away with water – the action is very gentle and the water helps to soothe and hydrate. Tissues can be harsh on fragile skin and may not completely remove residue to keep skins spot free, although you can find moist towelettes that remove all traces of make-up in just one swipe.

The new-generation cleansers mean that old-school toners are no longer needed to sweep away the alkaline film left by some cleansers, but if you live in a hard water area you may need to rinse for a little longer to shift deposits of water's naturally occurring minerals, such as calcium and magnesium.

Psychological needs aside, improved circulation and a more radiant complexion are probably the best results of a hands-on water-based routine.

Toning

Not long ago the accepted beauty routine was to cleanse, tone and moisturize. However, with the advent of rinse-off cleansers, separate toners are becoming increasingly old-fashioned. When rich cold creams and milky cleansers were mainstream, a separate toner was essential for removing any greasy residue. However, new formulations are making the need for a toner a rarity rather than the norm.

There are two types of toner. The first, for oily skin, can be formulated with up to 70 per cent alcohol and/or exfoliating salicylic acid; astringents such as witch hazel; solvents such as resorcinol; as well as colourants and fragrances. The second, for normal-to-dry skin, contains no alcohol and no other solvents but it does contain emollients such as allantoin or glycerine, soothing plant extracts and fragrances instead. Ultimately, unless you have a very oily skin or use a cleansing oil, milk or cold cream that does not rinse well, there is little need for either.

Toners can feel very refreshing but they are an alternative to water for removing excess oil. Unlike water, however, they can irritate the skin. Toners, astringents, clarifying lotions, refreshing mists and the like all contain solvents, which essentially dissolve and remove essential lipids from the skin's surface. If your skin is very dry, these solvents will cause your skin to dehydrate. So use toners cautiously and be guided by the reaction of your skin.

Hydrating

With the beauty focus now falling on added extras – antioxidants, fruit acids and sun protection – there's a tendency to forget that water is the basic common denominator, making up around 60 per cent of a typical skin-care product.

How do you know when a skin is thirsty? Dryness and tightness are the most obvious signs, but these are common to both dry and dehydrated skins – essentially two different conditions. Dehydrated skin may be naturally dry, normal or oily, but happens to be temporarily lacking in water. A good way to test for dehydration is to stand close to a mirror and move the skin of the cheek gently upward with the index finger. A dehydrated skin will fold into a tightly packed range of lines or ripples.

Taking in enough water, both externally and internally, is therefore crucial to preventing dehydration. When we become severely dehydrated, the skin's lower layer, which is 80 per cent water, 'donates' water to the rest of the body. Without water in the upper layer, enzyme activity slows down, skin becomes thinner, water evaporation accelerates and external aggressors penetrate easily.

If skin is not treated immediately, the skin deteriorates quickly, becoming fragile and irritated. The only way to break the cycle is to provide the skin with intensive, long-lasting hydration and to stimulate enzyme activity with an effective moisturizer.

A product's moisturizing abilities are also determined by the humectants it contains. These work by either drawing water up from the depths of the dermis or attracting it from the surrounding atmosphere. Look for hyaluronic acid, sodium PCA, propylene, butylene glycol or marine extracts.

Protecting

Given all that we know about the damaging effect of the sun, you need to protect your skin not only at the beach, beside the pool or in the great outdoors, but every time you go into the sun. While it's true that the darker your skin, the more protection you have against the sun's damaging rays, specialists warn that all skin tones are at risk for skin cancer, pigmentation, vision damage, and rapid ageing.

YOUR BEAUTY ROUTINE

One of the keys to beautiful skin is a cleansing routine that is gentle, thorough and relaxing.

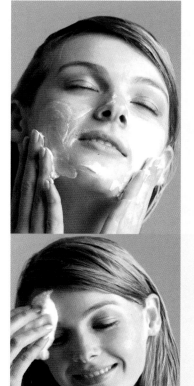

Pull hair back. Squeeze a walnut-sized blob of cleanser into your palm and gently warm it by rubbing it between your hands. This will emulsify the cleanser, making it more able to loosen dirt and grime.

Apply the cleanser with your fingertips, beginning at the centre of your face and working upwards and outwards. Massage the cleanser in with your fingertips to soften any congested areas in the skin. This relaxes the pores for further treatment and helps boost circulation. Rinse off excess cleanser.

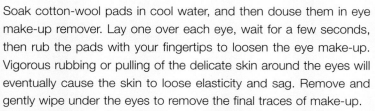

Soak cotton-wool pads in cool water, and then douse them in eye make-up remover. Lay one over each eye, wait for a few seconds, then rub the pads with your fingertips to loosen the eye make-up. Vigorous rubbing or pulling of the delicate skin around the eyes will eventually cause the skin to loose elasticity and sag. Remove and gently wipe under the eyes to remove the final traces of make-up.

Using cotton-wool pads soaked in warm water and alcohol-free toner, sweep the rest of the face to remove the cleanser. Gently splash with cool water to stimulate the skin before applying mask.

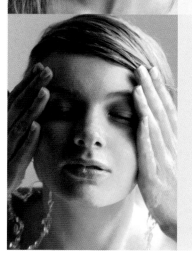

Apply the face mask, taking care to avoid the eye and lip areas. Don't forget your neck, which must be included in each and every step of the cleansing routine.

Remove the mask gently with a wet face cloth. Using clean cotton-wool pads soaked in warm water to remove any remaining traces, splash face and finish off with your moisturizer.

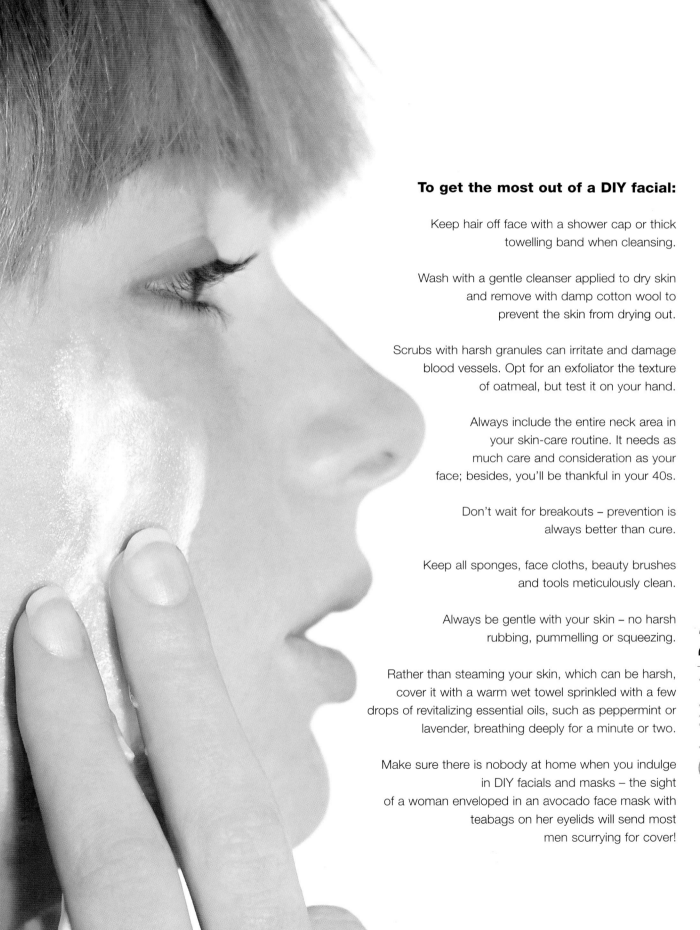

To get the most out of a DIY facial:

Keep hair off face with a shower cap or thick towelling band when cleansing.

Wash with a gentle cleanser applied to dry skin and remove with damp cotton wool to prevent the skin from drying out.

Scrubs with harsh granules can irritate and damage blood vessels. Opt for an exfoliator the texture of oatmeal, but test it on your hand.

Always include the entire neck area in your skin-care routine. It needs as much care and consideration as your face; besides, you'll be thankful in your 40s.

Don't wait for breakouts – prevention is always better than cure.

Keep all sponges, face cloths, beauty brushes and tools meticulously clean.

Always be gentle with your skin – no harsh rubbing, pummelling or squeezing.

Rather than steaming your skin, which can be harsh, cover it with a warm wet towel sprinkled with a few drops of revitalizing essential oils, such as peppermint or lavender, breathing deeply for a minute or two.

Make sure there is nobody at home when you indulge in DIY facials and masks – the sight of a woman enveloped in an avocado face mask with teabags on her eyelids will send most men scurrying for cover!

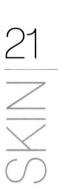

THE BASICS

Cream cleansers make light work of lifting make-up and impurities, and are ideal for use at night. Massage into the skin in small circular motions, and leave for a few seconds to dissolve impurities. Remove with damp cotton wool or moistened sponge.

Wash-off cleansers or pH-balanced soaps are ideal for use in the bath or shower. Together with facial cleansing brushes, these allow you to exfoliate and cleanse in one go.

Night creams are good investments when the skin's recuperative powers are at their height – from 23.00 to 01:00. They contain special ingredients to help the skin recover.

Moisturizers used daily are essential for all skin types. Look for formulations that contain a sunscreen, as well as antioxidants to prevent premature ageing, and sufficient hydration to suit your skin type.

Eye make-up removers are essential for cleansing the delicate eye area. Don't think you can use normal cleansers in this area – look for a gentler formulation, ideally containing no oil or fragrance. Work gently from the outer corner of the eye, taking care not to drag or pull the skin.

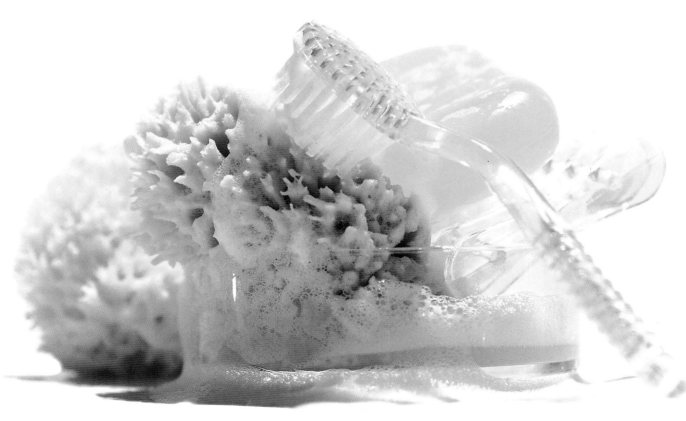

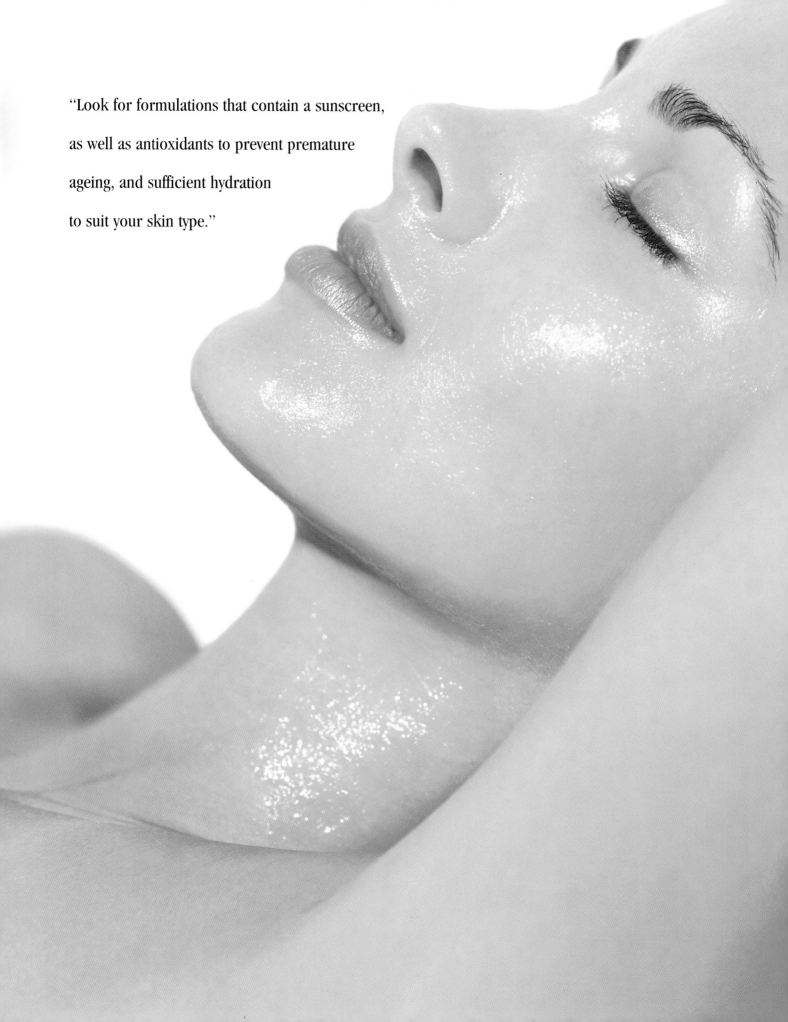

"Look for formulations that contain a sunscreen, as well as antioxidants to prevent premature ageing, and sufficient hydration to suit your skin type."

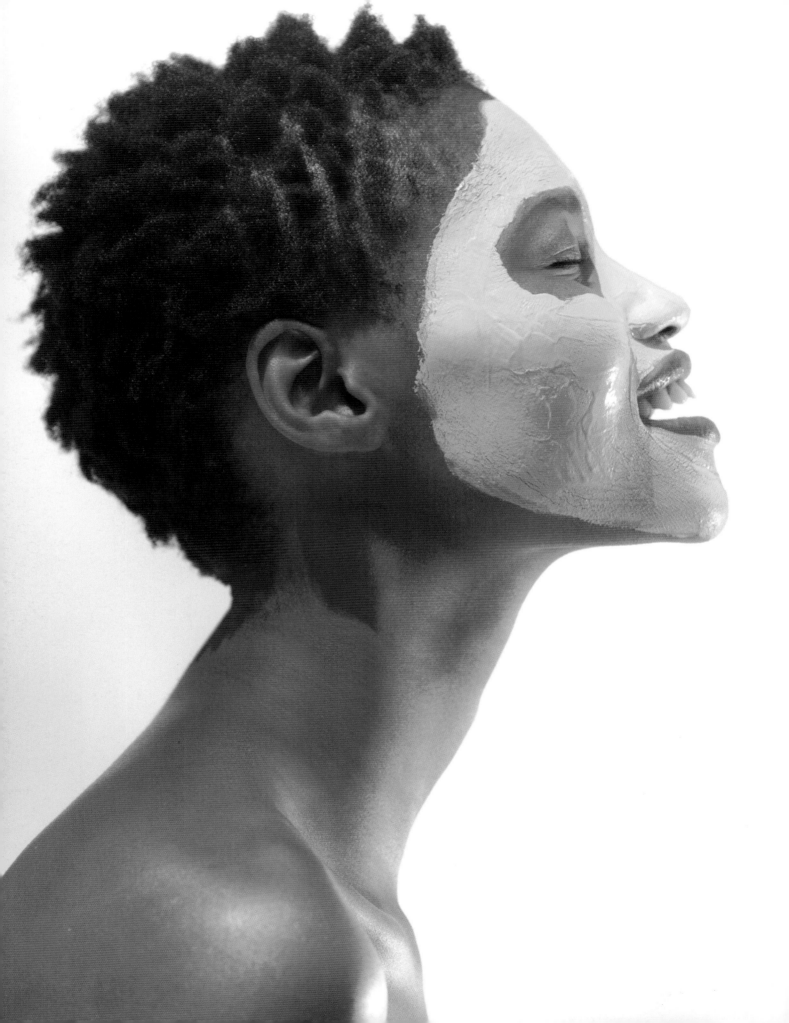

BEYOND THE BASICS

Cleansing, moisturizing and sun screening may be the mainstay of good skin care but cosmetic counters are filled to capacity with all sorts of other skin-care products – from masks and exfoliators to serums and eye creams. So how do these products fit into a sound beauty routine?

Masks

Face masks are considered more of a luxury than a necessity, but they infuse the skin with beneficial ingredients and offer a quick, albeit termporary, way to exfoliate, moisturize, cleanse or soothe.

Choose a mask formulated for your skin type. A clay mask can dry out and further irritate dry skin, while a moisturizing mask could aggravate acne-prone skin. If a mask stings, remove it immediately, unless you are using an AHA or BHA product where a mild tingling is not unusual.

Exfoliators

Exfoliators are essential for sloughing off dead skin cells. Use once a week to boost circulation. Dead cells and dirt sit on the surface, clogging pores, and make your complexion look dull.

However, moderation is the key. The top layer of the stratum corneum defends the skin, so you don't want to strip it. Avoid physical exfoliators like sponges, brushes, and loofahs – they are generally too abrasive and provide a breeding ground for bacteria. Also avoid cream-based exfoliators that are abrasive; the formulations should feel gentle on the skin.

Chemical exfoliators don't require rubbing and rinsing. For example, alpha-hydroxy acids (AHAs) dissolve the protein bonds that bind dead skin cells together, allowing you to shed the cells easily. If your skin tolerates AHAs, this is the best way to control the level of exfoliation. When it comes to exfoliating, more is not better! If you notice pink or raw patches on your skin, you know you've overdone it.

Eye creams

Eye creams are usually lighter in texture than most facial moisturizers and specially formulated not to harm the eye's delicate tissue. However fragrance, emulsifiers, and emollients are not uncommon and may cause sensitivity in the ultra-sensitive eye area.

For daywear choose a formula enriched with UV protectors and antioxidants. Gently pat into the skin under the eyes and along the orbital and brow bones. The skin's warmth helps to deliver it where it's needed. Avoid applying the product too close to the eyes. If it enters the tear duct it can aggravate the mucous membranes and cause puffiness.

Serums

Today's serums are usually a cocktail of potent but lightweight, anti-ageing ingredients. Some are designed to be used every day, others when your skin needs to generate new cells or deliver a burst of radiance. They are usually worn underneath your moisturizer, and many brands have cult followings.

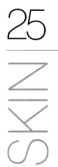

SKIN PROBLEMS

Decode your skin's SOS signals. Here's how to rescue skin in distress:

Skin changes to take to a doctor

While you can learn to read and respond to certain skin signals on your own, the following demand a doctor's attention:

- Sore or bleeding bumps that don't heal within a month
- Moles that change colour, size or shape
- Inexplicable blisters that itch or burn
- Any sudden, persistent or unexplained swelling.

Sensitive skin

This troublesome condition affects every type of skin in the form of redness, scaling, swelling and irritation. Skin can react to skin-care products and detergents just as it can to the sun, wind and pollution.

Do
- Use a sunscreen containing titanium dioxide
- Wash your face with lukewarm, not hot, water
- Use a fragrance-free moisturizer
- Try products that contain anti-inflammatories like camomile
- Use a liquid or gel cleanser low in detergent; the label should say 'pH balanced' or 'non-alkaline'.

Don't
- Use scented products
- Use astringents or toners that contain alcohol
- Use abrasive facial scrubs
- Smoke, it accelerates loss of elastin and collagen
- Steam or apply ice to the skin
- Use soap bars and bar cleansers
- Use skin-care products that contain preservatives like lanolin and mineral oil.

Stinging is a sign that a product is irritating your skin. It usually occurs immediately, so it's easy to identify the culprit. If you're using a potent anti-ageing product, ask for something gentler.

Itching may be an allergic reaction to a medication, cosmetic or skin-care product. Apply cold compresses and try to track down the source.

If your eyelids are itchy, you may have a contact allergy to latex or nickel in your eyelash curler or to formaldehyde in your nail polish.

If your hairline is itchy, red and scaly, your shampoo, conditioner, or hair colour may be responsible. The scalp is fairly resistant but the hairline, ears, and neck are not. Discontinue use.

Blackheads, also known as comedones, occur when sebum dries and hardens before it reaches the surface, blocking the pore in the process. When the sebum and dead cells in the follicle oxidize, they turn dark in colour.

Acne is thought to be triggered by hormonal changes that occur during puberty and times of stress. When this happens, levels of androgen rise and the sebaceous glands go into overdrive. This results in excessive amounts of oil, which ultimately lead to acne. The occasional spot is usually the result of bacteria penetrating the skin and causing infection.

Hyperpigmentation – or sun, age, brown or liver spots – are caused by an excess of melanin, the pigment that gives the skin its colour. Discontinue birth-control tablets or oestrogen-replacement pills and start using sunscreens.

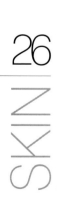

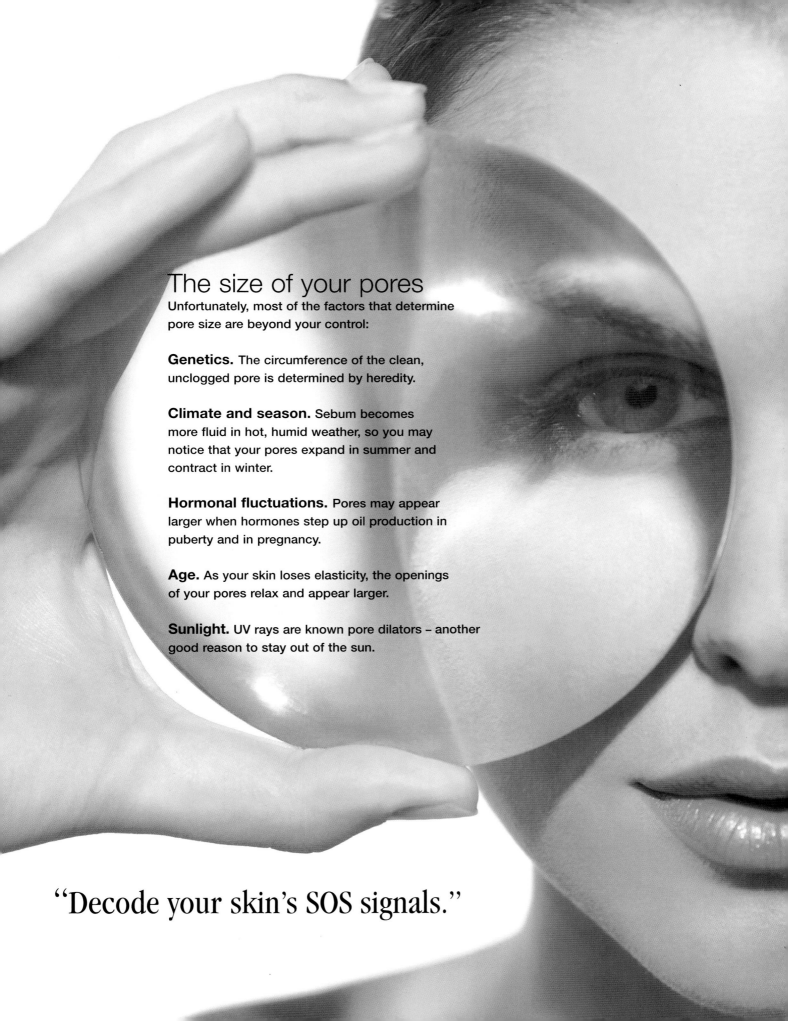

The size of your pores

Unfortunately, most of the factors that determine pore size are beyond your control:

Genetics. The circumference of the clean, unclogged pore is determined by heredity.

Climate and season. Sebum becomes more fluid in hot, humid weather, so you may notice that your pores expand in summer and contract in winter.

Hormonal fluctuations. Pores may appear larger when hormones step up oil production in puberty and in pregnancy.

Age. As your skin loses elasticity, the openings of your pores relax and appear larger.

Sunlight. UV rays are known pore dilators – another good reason to stay out of the sun.

"Decode your skin's SOS signals."

SPECIAL TREATMENTS

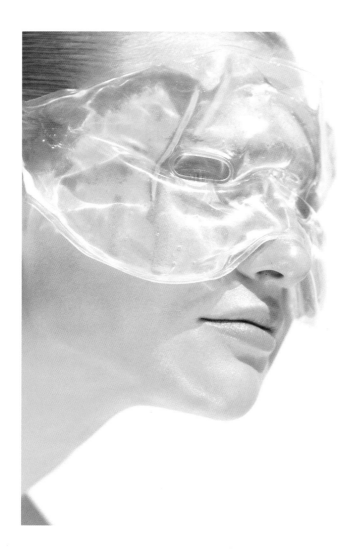

The skin's horny layer or stratum corneum is basically a graveyard for dead skin cells. Every 28 days or so, skin cells called keratinocytes migrate from the lowest level of the epidermis to the stratum corneum to die, forming a shield that keeps out harmful substances and helps block moisture loss.

So it makes sense to entrust the care of such a vital organ to a facial therapist. Even people with a normal skin are advised to wait four weeks between facials (for the full keratinization process) simply because too much of anything can irritate the skin. Anyone with inflamed acne, redness, pimples, or enlarged blood vessels should rather consult a dermatologist.

A typical facial at a salon will consist of cleansing, exfoliation, massage, extraction, and moisturizing. Ideally, skin type dictates treatment. For example, someone with oily skin will get an oil-absorbing mud mask, while someone with dry skin will have a facial massage with a rich moisturizer. So before laying a hand on you, an aesthetician should examine your skin carefully.

Most therapists report a substantial improvement in the texture and condition of the skins they treat. This is partly because an expert eye and a different pair of hands will be able to assess and treat problem areas more easily than you could yourself. The benefits aren't just restricted to your face – an hour in a beauty salon is a relaxing experience that relieves stress and gives your whole system a boost.

While you are having your facial, ask the beautician what she is doing, which products she is using and which she thinks will work for you. Look out for tips that you can use at home. Finally make a mental note of how your skin feels and looks after the facial to learn from the treatment.

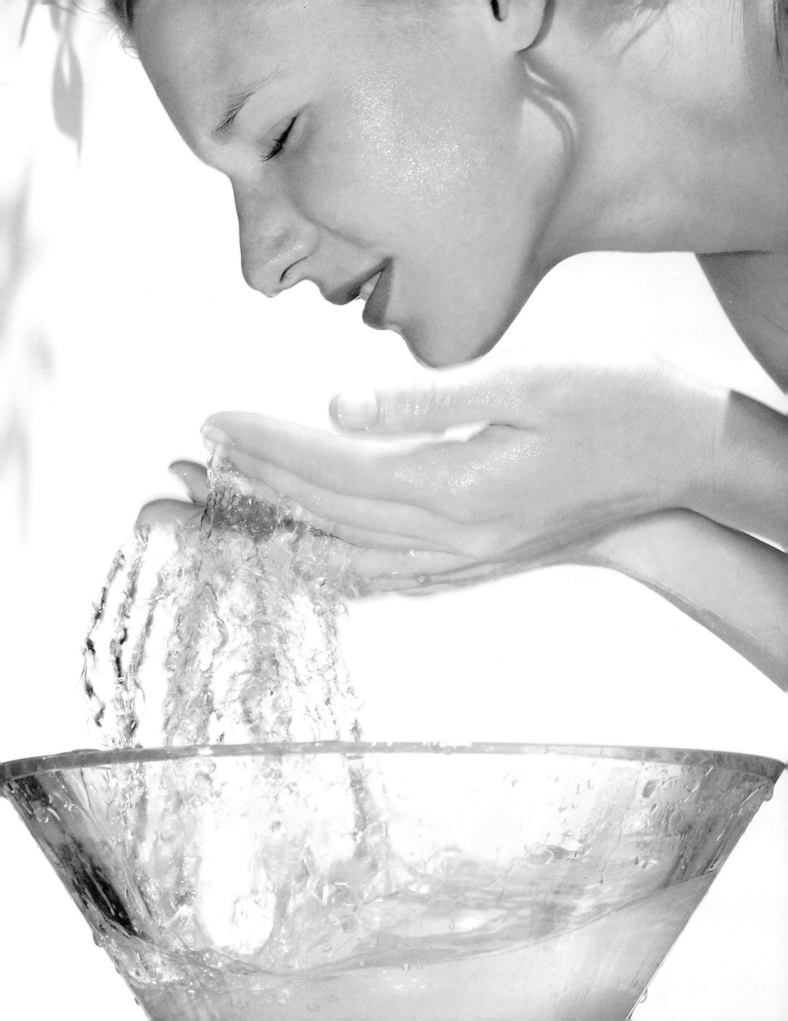

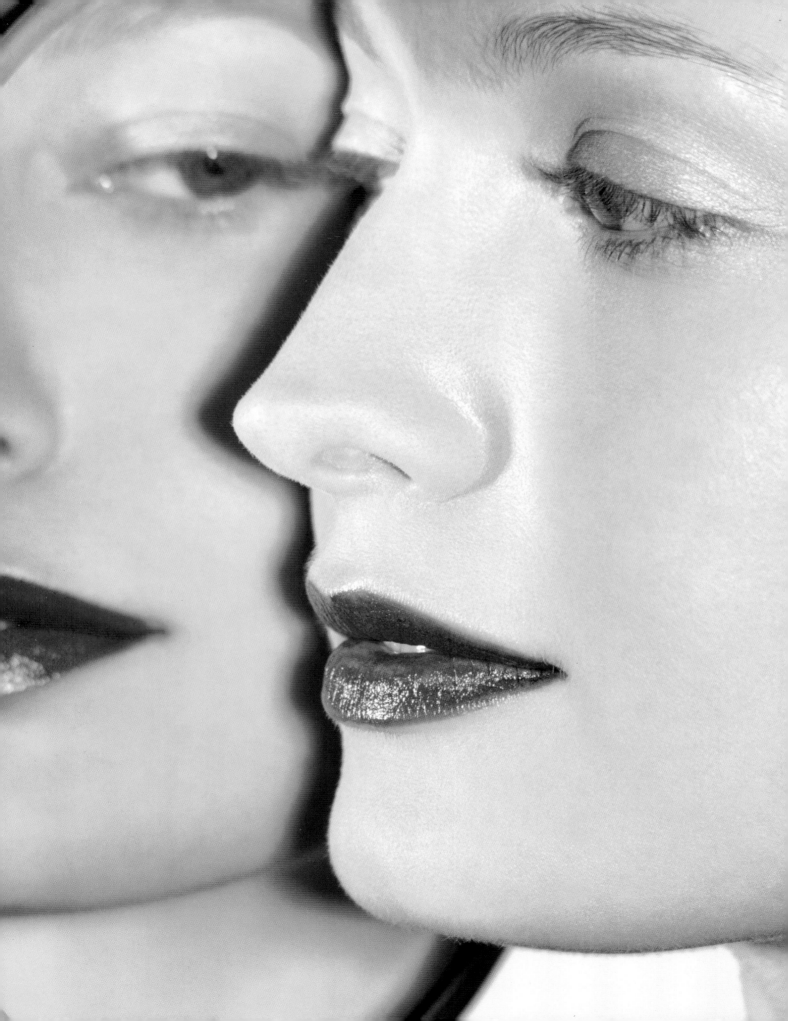

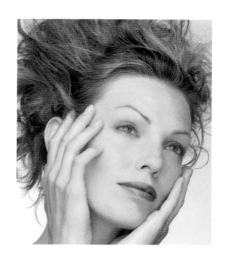

Everything in our body changes as we get older, and our skin is no exception. But the truth is, it's the way we treat our skin that 'ages' facial skin the most. Scientists explain this by saying there are two main types of ageing: intrinsic and extrinsic ageing. To understand the difference between the two, you need only look at the skin on your face versus, say, the skin on your hips or upper thighs. The prime cause of extrinsic ageing? Sun exposure.

ANTI ageing

"UV rays and pollution speed up the ageing process because they promote the production of free radicals."

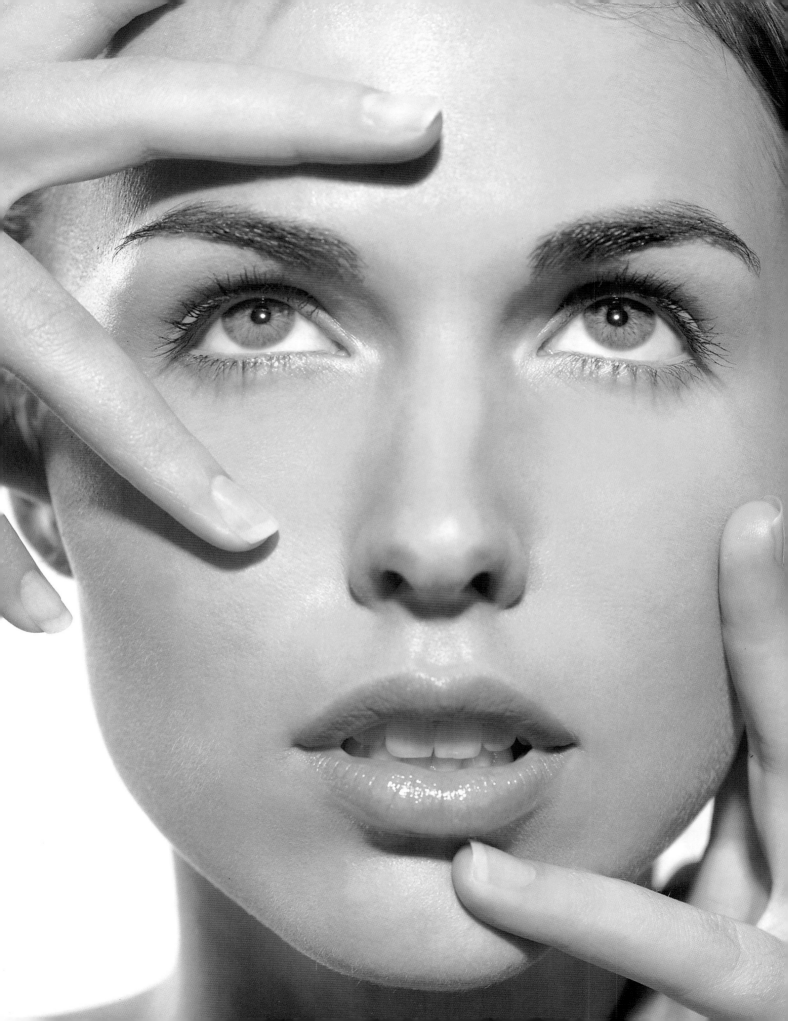

HOW WE AGE

Intrinsic ageing or chrono-ageing is the natural, biological ageing that occurs in the skin without sun damage and we have little control over it. Although a healthy diet, regular exercise, plenty of fresh air and tackling stress will certainly help, your skin will follow this inevitable ageing process:

- **Dryness.** The sweat glands and the oil glands are less productive after age 30, and the loss continues with time. This causes dry, wrinkled and itchy skin.
- **Loss of skin tone.** Pigment-producing melanocytes begin to burn out from your late 30s, producing paler, less radiant skin. They're also less able to fight sun damage, so uneven pigmentation is possible.
- **Thinning.** At around age 40, the dermis and the skin's fat layer start to get thin, making the skin more fragile and likely to abrade. The process picks up steam after your 50th birthday, and at 80 your skin is 30 per cent thinner than it was at 18. The unhappy result of this process: sagging and loss of plump, youthful softness.
- **Loss of elasticity and firmness.** Fibroblasts lose their ability to function over the years, reducing the production of collagen and elastin. There is also a general loss of muscle tone and a relocation of the fat under the skin's surface, resulting in flaccidity and a parchment-like appearance to the skin.
- **Diminished immune response.** The skin is home to Lagerhan's cells, receptors for the immune system that register the presence of foreign agents and toxins. When these grow old or are damaged by UV rays, you are less likely to get quick warning signals when you come in contact with irritants.
- **Reduced ability to repair damage.** Overall, the body loses its ability to repair free-radical damage, so changes in the cells become more pronounced.
- **Loss of temperature control.** As the sweat glands lose their ability to function, your body finds it harder to register heat and cold and to regulate itself.

Extrinsic ageing or photo-ageing, was until quite recently believed to be a fast-forwarding of intrinsic ageing. But differences between the damaging effect of the sun, air pollution, and inflammation caused by harsh detergents and rough treatment have emphasized the fact that external elements play a large part in the ageing process. In fact a staggering 80 per cent of skin ageing is attributed to sun damage.

UV rays and pollution (including smoking) speed up the ageing process because they promote the production of free radicals on the surface of exposed skin, damaging collagen and elastin fibres. The result is a rough, dry skin texture, deep wrinkles, uneven pigmentation and broken veins.

Hormonal ageing relates to lower levels of oestrogen in women as they mature. We see the following:

- A diminishing thickness and degradation of the natural processes that maintain epidermal hydration
- Age spots or seborrhoeic keratoses (brownish, sometimes raised spots) after menopause
- Sun spots or solar keratoses on the backs of hands and face
- Pale brown blotches during pregnancy, which are aggravated by sunlight
- Visible veins and even broken capillaries as the skin thins and hot flushes appear during menopause.

AGE PREVENTION

Don't fast forward

How we age is dependent on two factors: lifestyle and genes. If your parents aged well, then you will probably carry on looking good for a long time too. But how we live, even where we live, can also have a major impact on how we age. Here's how some lifestyle factors can add years, even decades, to our faces:

- Sunbaking or regular use of a sunbed – add 20 years! According to an increasing number of dermatologists, sunbeds are even more damaging to the skin than direct sunlight, because they emit pure UVA rays, which penetrate deep into the skin, causing long-term damage. Avoid entirely.

- Stress – add three years! A major skin ravager along with the excessive alcohol, caffeine consumption, missed sleep and skipped meals that accompany it. Try to reduce stress by finding new ways to relax and slow down.

- Crash dieting – add 10 years! Yo-yo dieting deprives your skin of vital nutrients. If you loose weight quickly, your skin will also stretch and sag.

- City living – add five years! Try a skin cream rich in antioxidants to clear up the damage.

The ageing process also gets a tremendous push from poor nutrition, cigarette smoke, harsh soaps, detergent-based moisturizers, excess alcohol and lack of sleep.

Get some sun sense

- Stay out of the sun between 11:00 and 15:00, even if it's overcast.
- The sun's intensity is the same wherever you are, so apply sunscreen before going out, and reapply frequently if you're swimming, exercising or perspiring.
- Dry off thoroughly after swimming. Drops of water have a 'magnifying glass' effect, and can intensify sunburn.
- Look beyond the SPF (sun protection factor). Not all sunscreens offer UVA protection.
- Wear SPF while driving because UVA rays penetrate glass.
- Wear bigger sunglasses to protect the whole eye area.
- Buy new sun-care products; the use-by date is usually only one year.
- Form a habit of wearing sunscreen on your face and hands every day. Look for a light sun-block you can wear under your make-up, or for a moisturizer that contains an SPF of 15.

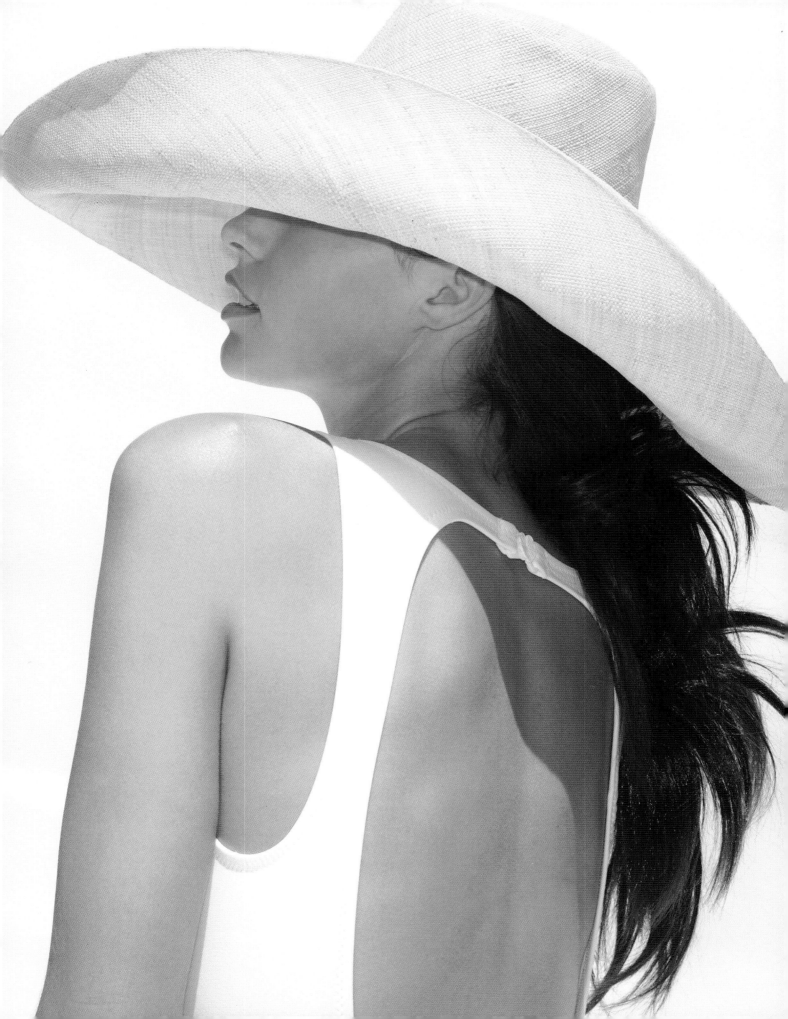

Signs of the times

at 20

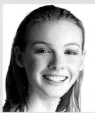

- Cells renew swiftly, blood circulates well, collagen and elastin are in peak form.
- At this stage, skin is usually self-sufficient, which means that it will be more prone to abuse – either through abrasive products or neglect.
- Roughness and dullness associated early sun damage.
- Mild pigmentary changes.
- Fine lines around the eyes.
- Acne breakouts.

at 30

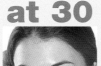

- Cell renewal and circulation slow down and skin starts to lose lustre.
- Expect a loss of plumpness as supportive collagen and elastin fibres weaken.
- An oily T-zone and adult acne can be triggered by stress, pregnancy and contraceptive or fertility drugs.
- Skin starts to sag; crow's feet, deeper smile and frown lines start to appear.
- Early sun exposure manifests as age spots. Uneven texture, rash-like acne rosacea and broken veins may appear.

at 40

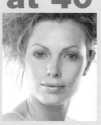

- Sebum production decreases and sensitivity increases.
- Deepened smile, frown, forehead, nose-to-mouth lines and crow's feet.
- More pronounced dehydration and sagging.
- Fine lines around the mouth increase as do sun-induced age spots.
- Oil glands get bigger and T-zone pores dilate.
- Years of sun damage may mean wrinkles, discoloration and broken capillaries.
- Circles under the eyes grow into pouches.

at 50

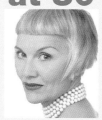

- Skin starts to acquire real character. Fine lines and wrinkles deepen into folds.
- Loss of elastin results in sagging skin.
- Menopausal changes can trigger acne.
- Signs of age show on the face, as well as the neck and hands.
- Skin tone becomes increasingly uneven with more age or sunspots.
- Increased sallowness, broken blood vessels and drier skin.

Carefully looking after your skin will stand you in good stead, but once the signs are in place, you'll want to see immediate results. So, plump the skin with moisturizer before applying make-up, avoid accentuating wrinkles by going easy on make-up, and keep everything as translucent as possible!

Professional treatment	What your skin needs
■ A regular facial will increase circulation and make your skin more receptive to products.	■ A regular beauty regime, a salon treatment every six weeks. ■ Apply serious sun protection at every opportunity and a moisturizer with at least SPF15 daily. ■ The eye area is the most vulnerable to early ageing, so now is the time to start using an eye cream. ■ Start extending your face cream right down your neck – you'll be thankful in your 40s.
■ A dermatologist can improve skin texture with retinol and glycolic peels. ■ Regular salon treatments are imperative to deep-cleanse and hydrate.	■ Thorough cleansing and facial massage increase circulation and make skin more receptive to products. ■ Most of your sun damage will have already occurred, but the effects of further damage still show in later years, so take cover with a protective moisturizer. ■ Use an exfoliator at least once a month.
■ Sun-induced age spots and acne can be treated by laser therapy or with glycolic acid. ■ Wrinkles can be softened and lips plumped with collagen and Botox injections.	■ Exfoliation and emolliation for throat and face are essential – the older you get the more you should exfoliate. ■ Choose milky or creamy cleansers, and keep toner to a minimum – don't imagine that toner closes pores, it doesn't. ■ Added extras include night creams and reviving face masks. ■ Use an eye gel in the morning if eyes are puffy and an eye cream for nourishment.
■ Laser, glycolic acid and Retin-A treatments become popular. ■ Botox injections cause a temporary paralysis of specific facial nerves.	■ Moisture and sun protection, essentially. ■ Time-fighting elements: collagen, elastin, and ceramides. An anti-ageing cream with vitamins A, C and E. ■ Added extras: fruit-acid night creams, hydrating masks, or firming day bases.

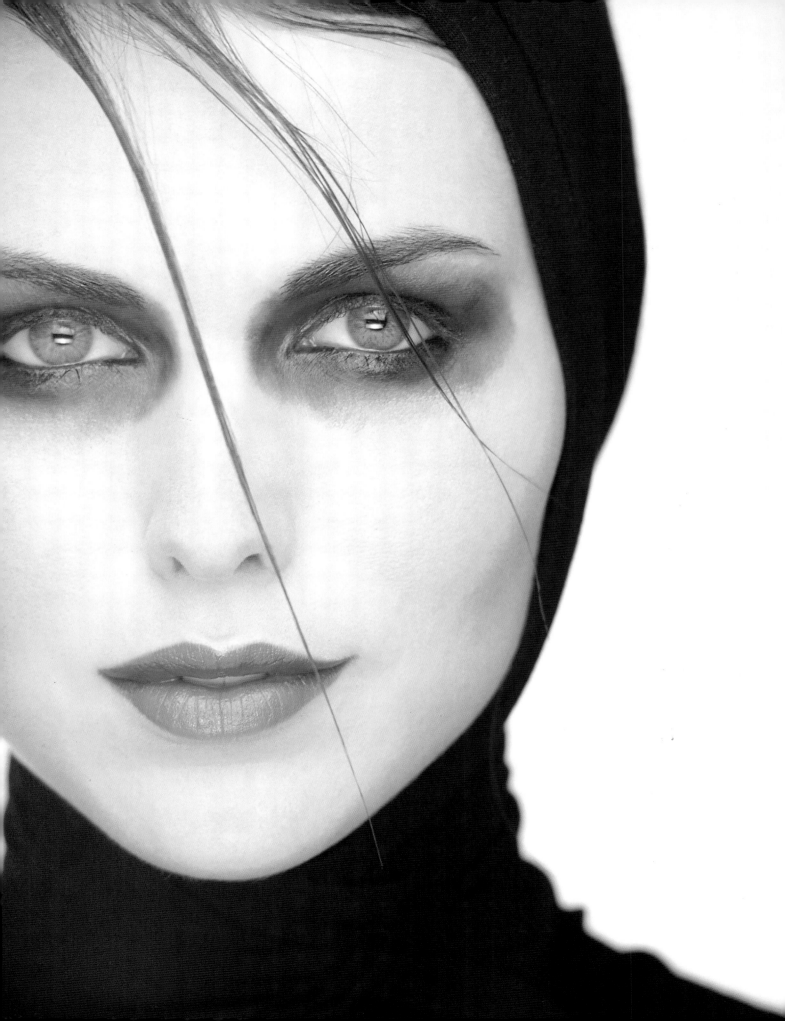

part two

the **power** of
MAKE-UP

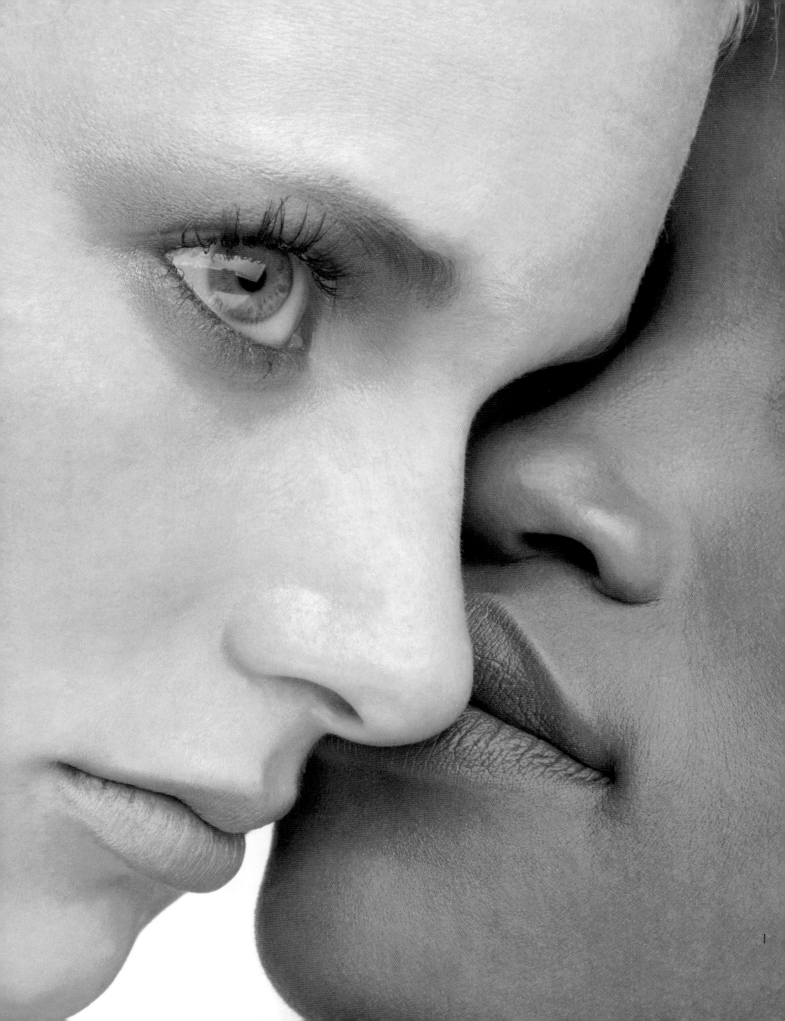

> **"Make-up is a way of expressing ourselves; it's about learning how to see ourselves differently. Try it out, what do you have to lose? You can always wash it off!"**

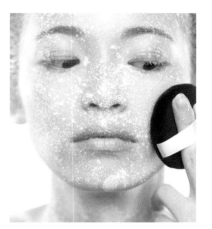

TOOLS
& techniques

Learn how to make your eyes stand out, make your lipstick last all day, minimize prominent jaws, create an even skin tone or higher cheekbones. Make-up is a way to celebrate those features we love and want to draw attention to.

Of course, with the cosmetic counters groaning under the weight of different textures and colour, actually deciding what you want to wear is far from easy. This probably explains why so many women are afraid to experiment with something new, especially colour.

Make-up is a way of expressing ourselves; it's about learning how to see ourselves differently. Try it out, what do you have to lose? You can always wash it off! Once you get the hang of it, make-up will make your confidence soar!

BRUSHES

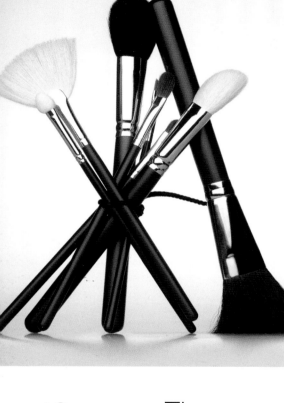

Investing in the right tools will make a tremendous difference in make-up application. Look for tools that feel good in your hand, that allow you to absorb and apply your product well. You already have the best tool of all – your fingertips, the perfect blenders. But to get into tight corners, nothing beats the precision of the right brush.

Your choice of brushes will have a lot to do with your style of applying make-up. If your application is elaborate and involves highlighting, contouring and many shades of eye shadow, you'll need a variety of brushes. If your make-up application is uncomplicated, you'll only need the basics.

When shopping for brushes look for sturdy handles and tightly anchored bristles. The basic kit should include five or six good-quality brushes. The ideal kit should include at least one slim eye-shadow brush, about 1.5cm (0.6in) thick, for the delicate lid, plus a slightly thicker one for blending.

A lip brush is brilliant for finishing off the last bits of your favourite lipstick but even better for lip definition. A blusher brush is essential: look for a firm, dome-shaped brush about 3cm (1.2in) in diameter. This will hold more colour at the centre and won't leave a harsh line.

An eyebrow brush with firm bristles controls the short brow hairs – an old toothbrush is ideal. A powder brush is good for fine application of powder, and finally an eyeliner brush should be a small, firm, flat brush for applying powder at the base of the eyelashes.

Tips

- Most brushes have either synthetic or natural bristles. Although modern synthetics are pretty good, nothing beats natural bristles for fine and transparent blending. Many professional make-up artists prefer sable brushes, which you can find at art supply stores.
- Test brushes before buying by brushing over your hand a few times to make sure that they don't shed too many bristles when you use them.
- Check that bristles are tightly packed. Cheaper brushes tend to have fewer bristles, loosely packed, and don't offer a long-term investment.
- Professional make-up companies offer the widest selection of brushes.
- Avoid stiff or hard brushes.
- Don't forget to knock the excess powder off the brush before you apply the colour to your face.
- Don't wipe or rub the brush across your face; instead, brush on with short, even strokes.

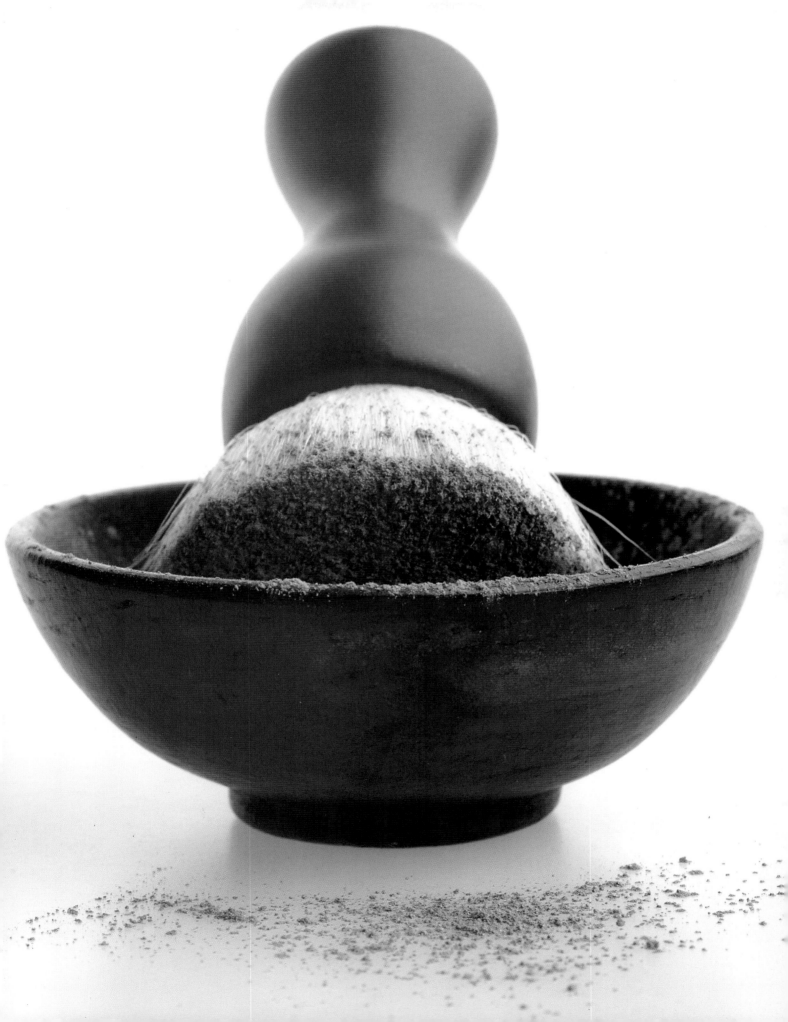

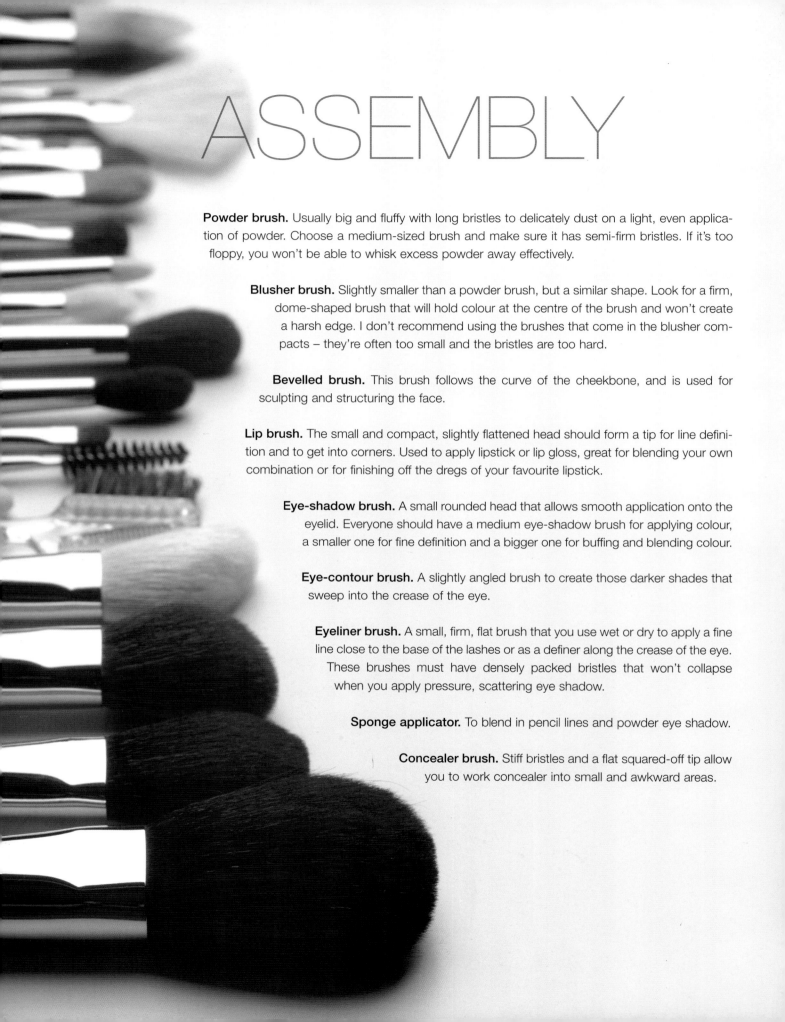

ASSEMBLY

Powder brush. Usually big and fluffy with long bristles to delicately dust on a light, even application of powder. Choose a medium-sized brush and make sure it has semi-firm bristles. If it's too floppy, you won't be able to whisk excess powder away effectively.

Blusher brush. Slightly smaller than a powder brush, but a similar shape. Look for a firm, dome-shaped brush that will hold colour at the centre of the brush and won't create a harsh edge. I don't recommend using the brushes that come in the blusher compacts – they're often too small and the bristles are too hard.

Bevelled brush. This brush follows the curve of the cheekbone, and is used for sculpting and structuring the face.

Lip brush. The small and compact, slightly flattened head should form a tip for line definition and to get into corners. Used to apply lipstick or lip gloss, great for blending your own combination or for finishing off the dregs of your favourite lipstick.

Eye-shadow brush. A small rounded head that allows smooth application onto the eyelid. Everyone should have a medium eye-shadow brush for applying colour, a smaller one for fine definition and a bigger one for buffing and blending colour.

Eye-contour brush. A slightly angled brush to create those darker shades that sweep into the crease of the eye.

Eyeliner brush. A small, firm, flat brush that you use wet or dry to apply a fine line close to the base of the lashes or as a definer along the crease of the eye. These brushes must have densely packed bristles that won't collapse when you apply pressure, scattering eye shadow.

Sponge applicator. To blend in pencil lines and powder eye shadow.

Concealer brush. Stiff bristles and a flat squared-off tip allow you to work concealer into small and awkward areas.

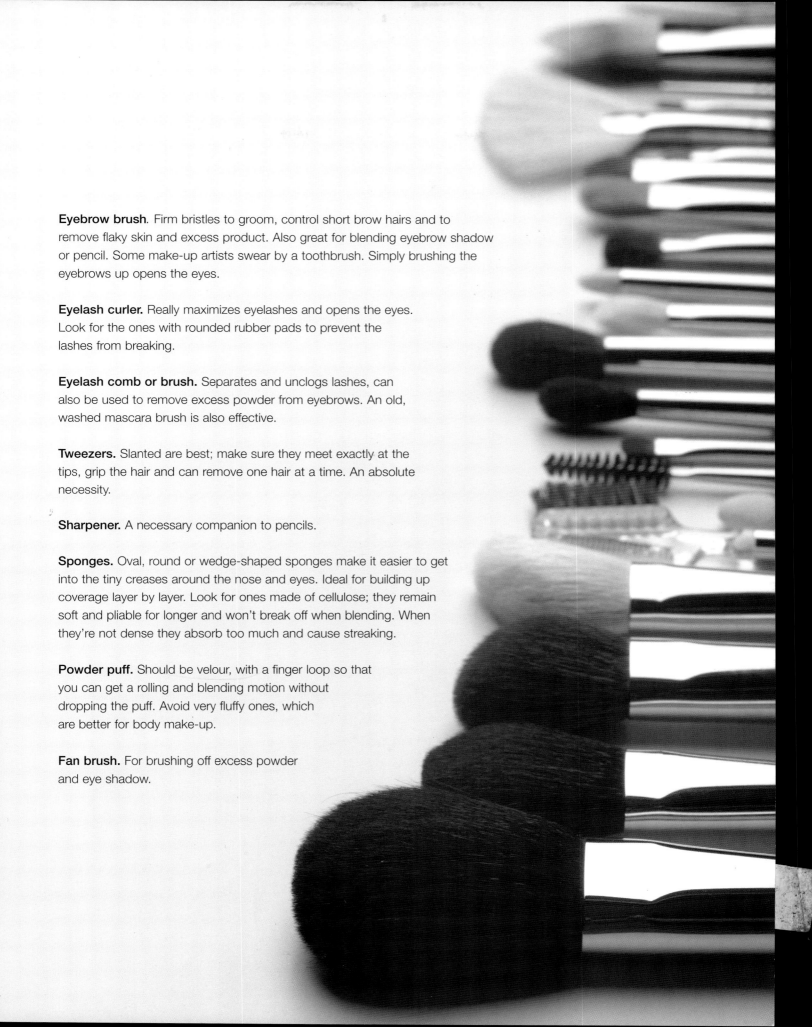

Eyebrow brush. Firm bristles to groom, control short brow hairs and to remove flaky skin and excess product. Also great for blending eyebrow shadow or pencil. Some make-up artists swear by a toothbrush. Simply brushing the eyebrows up opens the eyes.

Eyelash curler. Really maximizes eyelashes and opens the eyes. Look for the ones with rounded rubber pads to prevent the lashes from breaking.

Eyelash comb or brush. Separates and unclogs lashes, can also be used to remove excess powder from eyebrows. An old, washed mascara brush is also effective.

Tweezers. Slanted are best; make sure they meet exactly at the tips, grip the hair and can remove one hair at a time. An absolute necessity.

Sharpener. A necessary companion to pencils.

Sponges. Oval, round or wedge-shaped sponges make it easier to get into the tiny creases around the nose and eyes. Ideal for building up coverage layer by layer. Look for ones made of cellulose; they remain soft and pliable for longer and won't break off when blending. When they're not dense they absorb too much and cause streaking.

Powder puff. Should be velour, with a finger loop so that you can get a rolling and blending motion without dropping the puff. Avoid very fluffy ones, which are better for body make-up.

Fan brush. For brushing off excess powder and eye shadow.

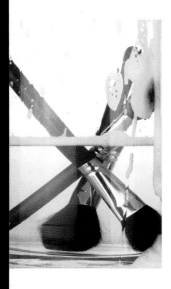

Clean-up acts

Beware the unwashed make-up brush. It will leave traces of unwanted bacteria and colour on your face and will hinder the application of powder, lipstick and concealer. Follow these hints to get the best out of your brushes:

- If you use make-up tools every day, wash them regularly every four to six weeks.
- Use a mild baby shampoo to clean brushes and rinse with a mild antiseptic solution.
- Never soak brushes or wet handles – wooden ones swell and lose bristles.
- For long powder brushes, sweep through shampoo diluted with tepid water, then rinse under tap.
- Finer brushes should be dipped into neat shampoo, then lathered before rinsing.
- Direct heat damages bristles, so don't blow dry with your hair dryer.
- To dry, carefully squeeze out excess water with a towel, reshape and lay brushes flat on the edge of the basin, allowing the air to circulate. Dry overnight.

Dirt alert

Bacteria thrive in neglected cosmetic jars, and most cosmetics have a limited shelf life. Unopened cosmetics remain stable for about three years, but a product may remain on a store shelf for a year before it gets to your cupboard.

Most cosmetic houses have sell-by dates or bar codes, but you should look at the cosmetics in the same way you would food to see if they have gone off. If the oil and pigment have started to separate, they are almost certainly past their sell-by date. Most are past their best after six months or so.

Usually, the drier a product, the longer it lasts. Microorganisms need water to grow, so creams and lotions are at high risk. Always try to use a pump applicator or tube; they're ideal for contamination-free application. Many jars now come with a spatula to keep out grubby fingers. If not, ask for one.

Hygiene tips

- Hygiene is an important aspect of make-up care. Wash your make-up bag itself every few weeks and rinse brushes, powder puffs and sponges in soapy water at least once a month.
- You are particularly at risk of infection in the case of mascaras and other products that come into contact with the eyes, so never be tempted to share or lend your make-up.
- Be careful when testing lipsticks; the herpes virus is easily transmitted via lipstick. Rather test lipsticks on the back of your hand.

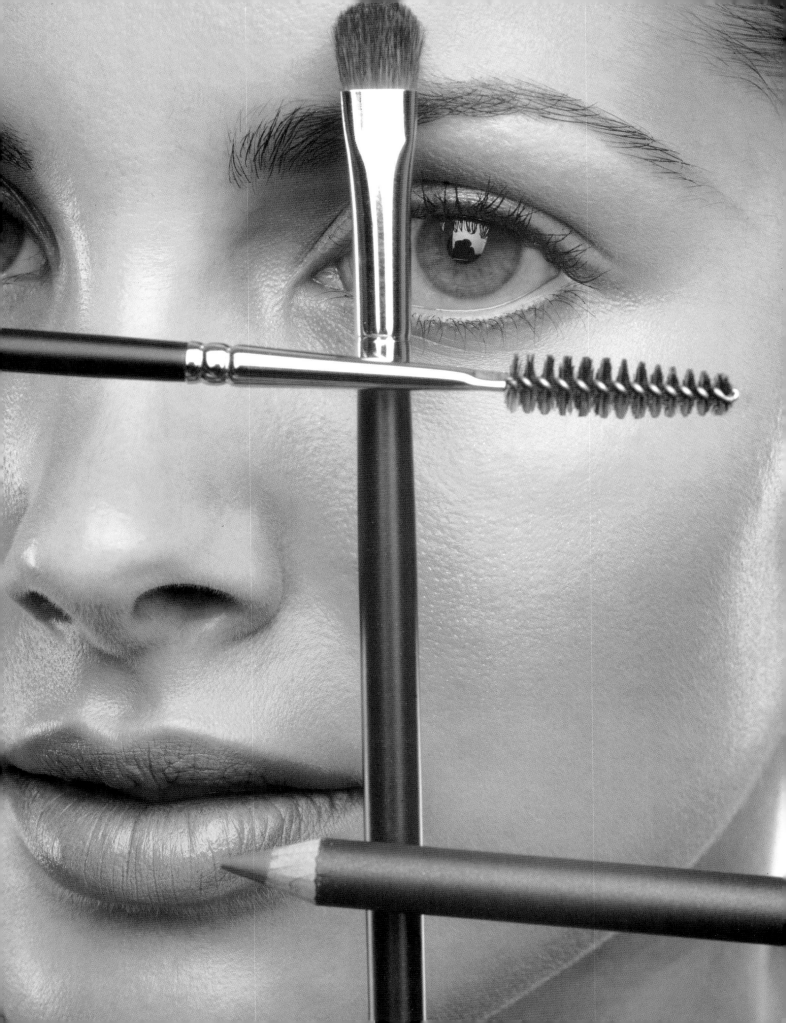

Palettes

Palettes are really only for the complete make-up junkie. Avoid the pre-packaged sets, or you'll land up with all sorts of colours that you never use. Look for options that you can customize your-self – the ideal palette should include two blusher options.

Palette tips

Blend lip colours together on the back of your hand or the lid of the palette before applying. It works better than applying one colour on the lips and then another, unless of course you're just applying a shimmer or gloss over the main colour.

A brown or burgundy lip colour will tone and transform any shade, even the garish ones. That's one good reason not to ditch those 'vibrant' mistakes.

It's also worth including a gloss, a shimmery gold or silver to make creamy colours look pearly, a classic blue-red to create dif-ferent shades of pink, and one of your favourite natural daytime colours.

Love lipstick variety?

Why not make a downscale version of a professional make-up artist's lip palette – a compact filled with decapitated lipsticks, squished into small moulds? This allows you to blend creatively and is also a good way to make use of worn-down lipsticks that can no longer be applied straight from the tube.

Professional make-up stores are the best place to source lipstick palettes – but there is a simpler and less expensive solution. Pop into an art supply store and look for a children's watercolour paint-box; prise out the watercolour blocks and rinse the palette to remove any paint remains. Then use a sharp knife to remove the remnants of each lipstick from its casing before patting the colours well down into moulds. Leave in a warm kitchen to help the colours settle. Don't pop into the microwave; some lipsticks contain metallic pigments, which will cause your palette to blister. Smooth over with a flat knife and then place in the fridge to harden.

Travel kits

Look for one of those multi-pocketed make-up rolls on a hanger. They are wonderful because you can store every item of skincare and make-up in the same place. Simply whip it out of your suitcase and hang it up in the bathroom as soon as you arrive at your destination for instant access.

Collect sample or trail-sized cosmetics for your travels – what better time to indulge in beauty treats than on holiday? Cabin-pressure wreaks havoc on your skin creams, and sharp climatic change has a detrimental effect on cosmetic products, so always try to decant your favourite items into plastic bottles before you board a plane.

To prevent bottles containing liquid from exploding mid-flight, create an airtight seal by squeezing the open bottles until the liquid reaches the top, and immediately close the cap tightly. For extra insurance, pack bottles in a plastic zip-loc packet and tape down the lid of anything creamy to prevent messy accidents in your luggage.

Pro kits

This is a great way to store all your make-up products, but pro kits are heavy to cart around. Look for a small version to organize and sort your products; what could be better than neatly ordered pull-out drawers of cosmetic products? Beats scratching around the bottom of a cosmetic bag.

Cosmetic bags

Look for transparent cosmetic pouches in different sizes, which will help you to find products in seconds and end those fruitless searches for missing items.

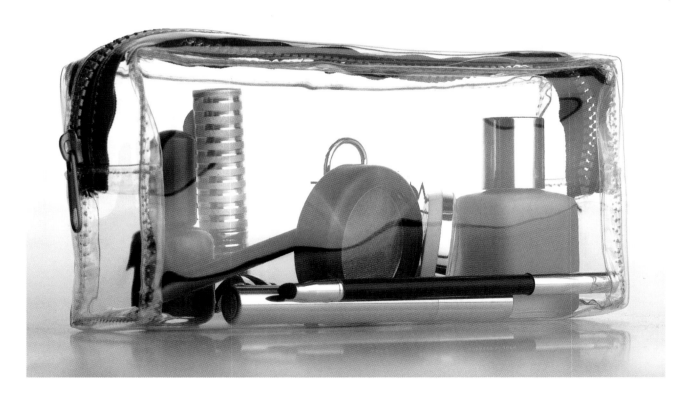

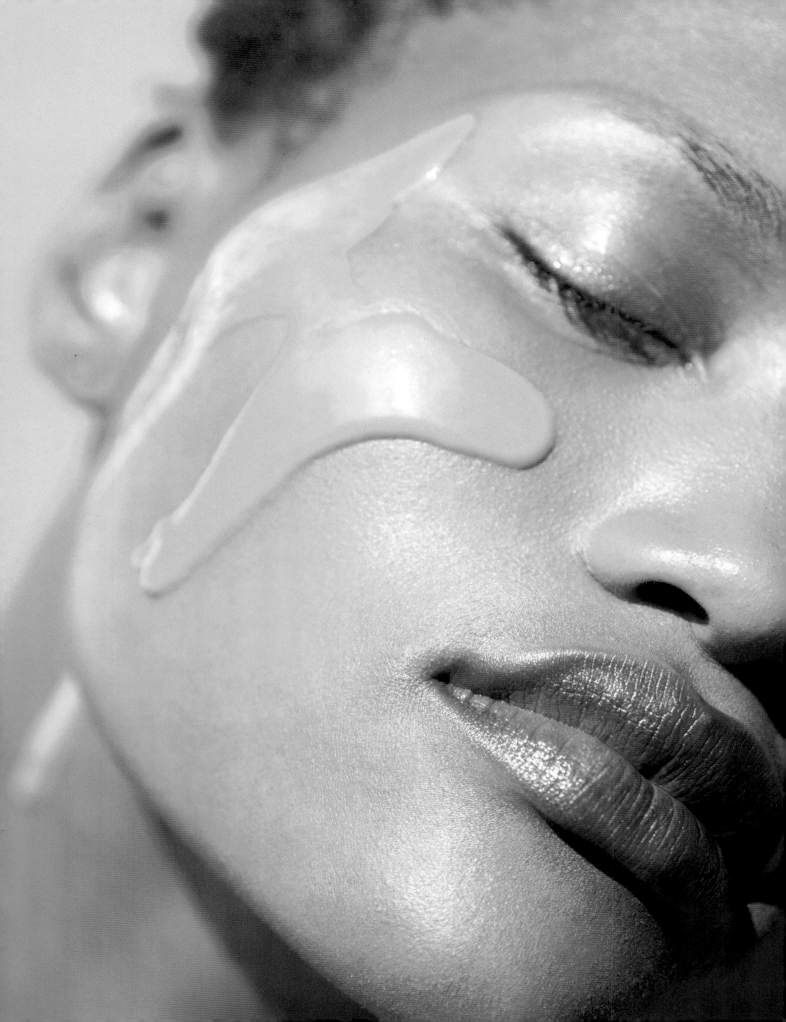

"Duplicate the look of perfect skin, rather than perfectly applied make-up."

FOUNDATION

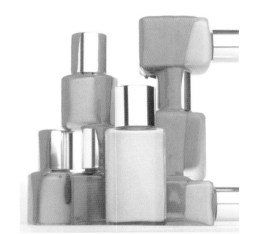

With new treatment benefits, sheer textures and believable colour, foundation is your skin's new best friend. Not so long ago if you asked for a foundation – that's what you got. Who cared if it looked unnatural, felt like cement, was 10 shades too light and blocked your pores? Everyone was wearing it!

Today this one-size-fits-all approach is thankfully outdated. Improved technology and heightened consumer awareness means that you can choose the shade, the texture and the amount of coverage, as well as a host of other skin-care benefits.

Cosmetic companies now see foundation as a natural extension of skin care: they protect your skin from the ageing effects of the sun and air pollution. Many come in variants that are suitable for oily, dry or sensitive skin – they can even balance combination skin and help fight acne.

MATCHING YOUR SKIN TYPE

Choose a product that suits your skin type and condition, not just your skin colour. There are formulations to suit everything from dry to oily and combination skins. Young skin needs less coverage and oil-free foundation, while mature, drier skin needs hydration. Remember that smooth, even-toned skin immediately looks younger. Consider added benefits like hydration, sun, and anti-ageing protection. Why not have flawless skin while fighting free radicals at the same time?

Added benefits

Some foundations offer a lot more than just coverage. Companies that put their money where their make-up is provide optional extras:

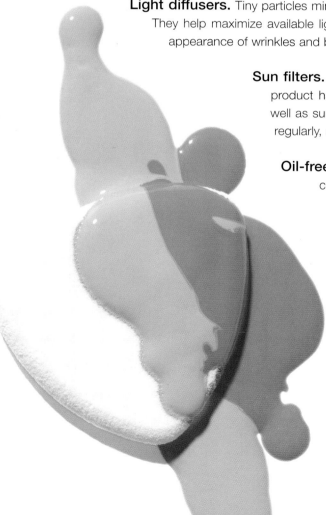

Light diffusers. Tiny particles minimize flaws by reflecting the light instead of absorbing it. They help maximize available light, reflecting a flawless complexion and diminishing the appearance of wrinkles and blemishes.

Sun filters. SPF 8 or higher gives some protection, but check that a product has UVA and UVB filters to prevent premature ageing as well as sunburn. To be fully effective, the base should be reapplied regularly, as with any other sunscreen.

Oil-free foundations. Special combination-skin foundations combine oil-absorbers with oil-free moisturizers for drier areas. Some acne-fighting formulas use salicylic acid, an exfoliant for break-out control. Look for non-comedo-genic, non-acnegenic formulas.

Skin-care. Bases may include salicylic acid to help exfoliate and to prevent outbreaks; oil inhibitors; antioxidant vitamins (usually C and E) to preserve the skin's elasticity; and hydrating agents.

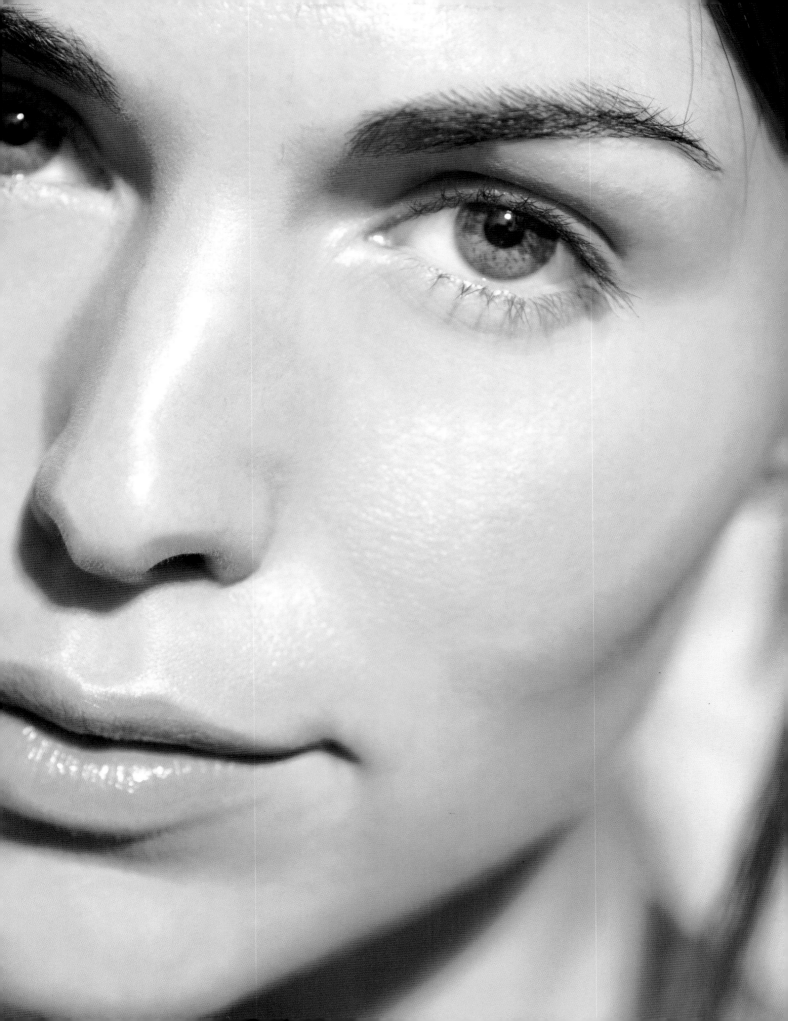

CHOOSING YOUR SHADE

When applied, foundation should seem to disappear completely into your skin. Your eye should not be able to discern the difference between your skin and the foundation. At the counter, smear a little along your jaw, then grab a mirror and check your face in daylight. If it's hard to see, it's the right shade. If it's obvious, go back and try again. Don't test foundation shades on your wrist; the jaw or neck are the best areas for a natural match.

The best foundations are now yellow-toned, which make-up artists have deemed to be the most universally skin-flattering colour. Never go for a darker shade in the hope that it will make you look more tanned and healthy. It's one thing to wear a tinted moisturizer, which is light and sheer, but the heavier texture of most foundations will be far more obvious. Not only will a darker shade look unnatural, it will also be almost impossible to blend at the edges.

Be careful to test your foundation in natural light, ideally in front of a window. Sometimes cosmetic counters use incandescent light that can make your skin look more yellow and golden than natural light. When shopping for foundation in a store, walk around and look at a test patch on your skin to make sure you are happy in a variety of lighting conditions.

Remember when wearing foundation, the final colour achieved is always a mix of your skin colour, the foundation colour, the foundation formula's coverage, the amount applied and the application method. So once you have discovered a shade that works for you, take the bottle with you to the cosmetic counter when you need a replacement; it'll help narrow the selection.

If you have black skin, you won't have to custom-blend as much as you did in the past. Nowadays cosmetic companies are constantly upgrading and adding more suitable shades and formulations for black skins. The only difference between white and black cosmetics is one of the main ingredients used to aid good coverage – titanium dioxide. Though used widely in Caucasian powders and foundations, it imparts a sallow, ashy appearance on black skins. Zinc dioxide has a similar effect and mica leaves a sparkly reflective finish, which can emphasize shine on black skins. Choose foundations without these ingredients as well as an oil-free formulation.

Shading tips

- To select the proper shade, test your foundation colour on the lower cheek area, just above the jawline. Select three foundation shades closest to your natural skin tone. Apply one at a time, allowing time for it to react with you skin's acid levels, then check the colour again in natural light. The one that seems to 'disappear' will be the correct shade.
- What looked right as a foundation base in mid-winter may look a little pale and insipid come the summer months, when you'll probably want a lighter texture and a subtler shade.

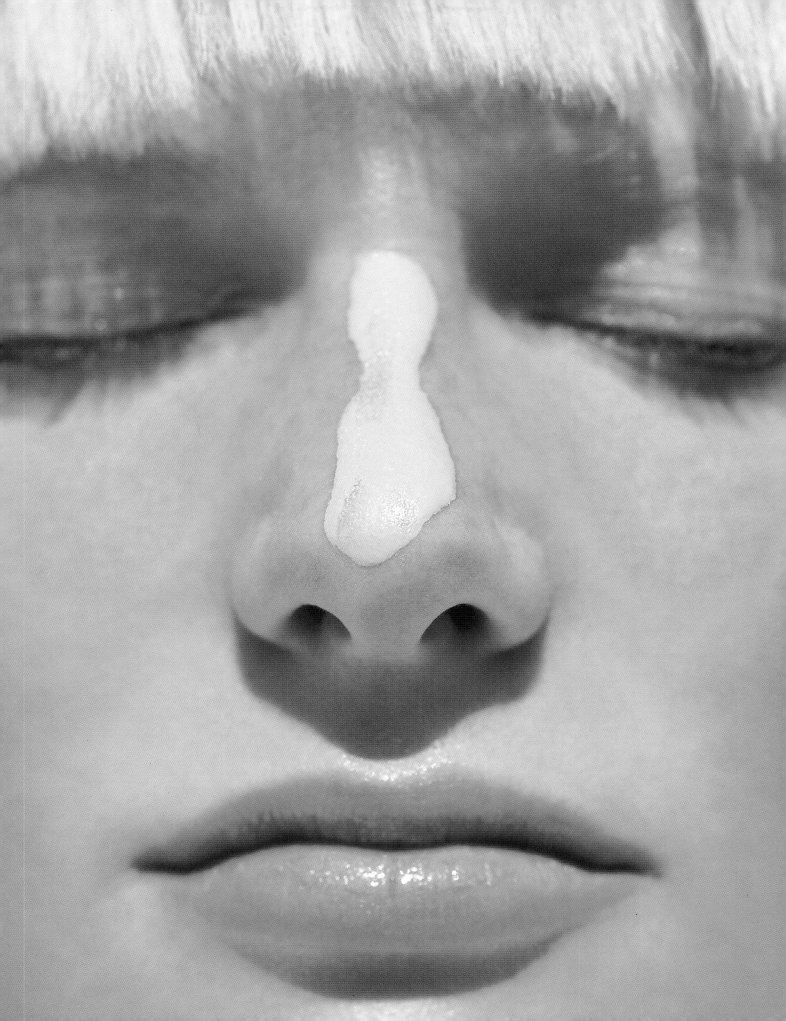

FINDING YOUR FORMULA

The perfect foundation suits your face and your lifestyle. Choose from one of these formulas:

Tinted moisturizers combine SPF, subtle coverage and hydration. Ideal for the natural, barely-there effect. the only catch is that they offer very little to no camouflage for blemishes.

Stick foundation can be used as foundation and concealer. Gives good coverage, but can be quite greasy, so avoid it if your skin is prone to oiliness. Ideal if you're on the move. Touching up is easy: if your colour matches perfectly, apply with fingers or use a dampened sponge for best results.

Compact foundation creates a completely natural look. Use sparingly for the sheerest cover.

Liquid foundation is easy to apply for complete coverage, but still looks natural. You can control the amount of coverage – make sure you blend carefully. Oily skins need oil-free formulas.

Powder foundation comes in a compact and provides light-to-medium coverage. It looks and acts like a pressed powder, but provides a little more coverage and can stay in place better than compact foundation. Ideal for oily skin because the powder helps absorbs oil. Apply wet or dry from the compact: perfect for touch-ups. Loose powder is best applied at home when you do your face in the morning.

Cream-to-powder foundations are a cross between pressed powder and creamy liquid foundation. The compact format means you can make up on the run with more coverage than pressed powder foundation; but they can look heavy and emphasize wrinkles, especially if your skin is prone to dryness. Apply with a dry sponge to give a matte finish, or use a damp sponge for a sheer look.

Added benefits

- **Light diffusers.** Tiny particles minimise flaws by reflecting light instead of absorbing it. Some foundations also introduce a buffer between the pigment and the skin by surrounding the pigment with moisturizing lipids, to prevent make-up from settling into fine lines.
- **Sun filters.** An SPF of 8 or higher gives some protection, but check that a product has UVA and UVB filters to prevent premature ageing as well as sunburn. Reapply regularly, as with other sunscreens.
- **Oil-free foundations.** Special combination-skin foundations combine oil-absorbers with oil-free moisturizers for drier areas. Some acne-fighting formulas use salicylic acid, an exfoliant to control breakout. Look for non-comedogenic or non-acnegenic foundations, or both.
- **Volatile silicones.** Aid the spread or slip of foundation and evaporate in seconds to leave a matte finish.
- **Skincare.** Bases may contain antioxidant vitamins (usually vitamin C and E) in order to preserve the skin's elasticity; and hydrating agents or oil inhibitors.

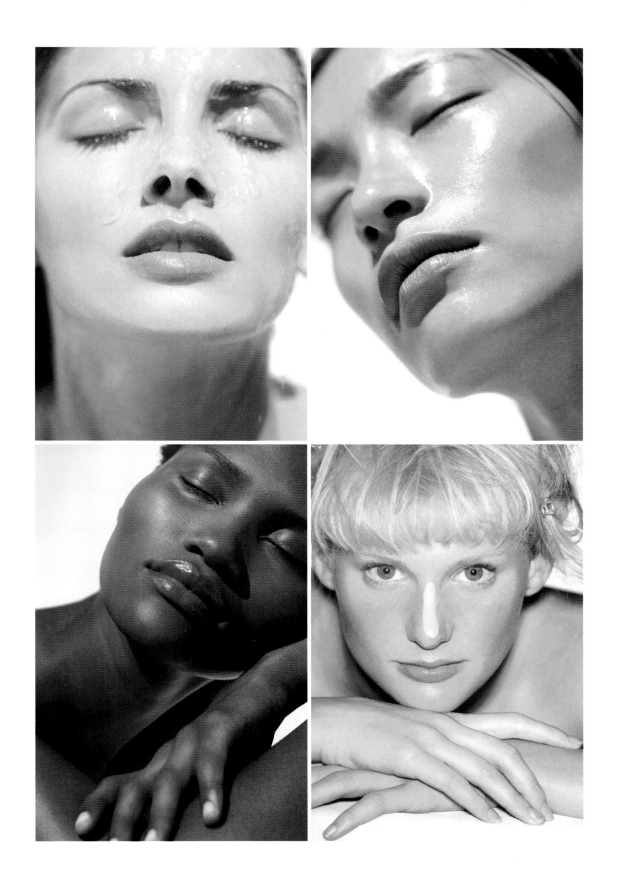

SEVEN STEPS TO PERFECTION

1 **Application.** Start with clean, well-moisturized skin, allowing the product time to sink in. Apply in daylight, ideally a north-facing window. For full-face coverage, dot foundation on the forehead, nose, chin and cheeks. If you want only partial coverage, just dab where needed. Finger application is idiot-proof, although a sponge is more hygienic. Start with a little, you can always add more.

2 **Blending.** Blend foundation using your fingers, pressing and patting lightly into the skin, and then if you like, a damp sponge for an even, sheer coat. Build up coverage with thin layers and ideally apply only where needed. A daytime application looks best if you still have freckles showing, cheeks blooming and a healthy glow. Always apply foundation downward, otherwise you'll accentuate pores and fine hairs. Apply over eyelids as a base for eye shadow. Remember to sweep over the ears and under the jaw, blending perfectly to avoid tide marks. Whisk off excess with a damp sponge if you overdo it.

3 **Concealer.** Using a small brush or your finger, dot concealer around the inner and outer corners of your eyes. Gently press and blend into skin with your ring finger but don't rub in, as this will 'drag' delicate under-eye skin. Best if you apply over your foundation, so that you can even out your skin tone.

4 **Cover up.** Hide any other blemishes that show through your foundation by dotting concealer with a sponge or small brush in tricky areas, such as under the jawline or around the nose. Pat it on with your finger to settle it on the skin.

5 **To set eye make-up.** To set concealer and foundation under and around the eyes, lightly dust them with a small, fine brush dipped in loose powder. Be careful not to apply too much; excess powder will only emphasize fine lines.

6 **To set foundation and concealer.** Use a translucent powder that complements your foundation and won't rob your skin of its natural glow, or a slightly yellow-toned powder to give skin warmth. With a large, round brush, dust a little over shiny areas. For a matte finish, gently press and roll a lightly powdered velour puff into your skin.

7 **Checks and balances.** Keep an eye on your make-up throughout the day. Use a lighter formulation in summer or carry a stick foundation for easy touch-ups. Avoid over-powdering if you don't want to look caked. For a matte finish, balance out with moist lips or eyes.

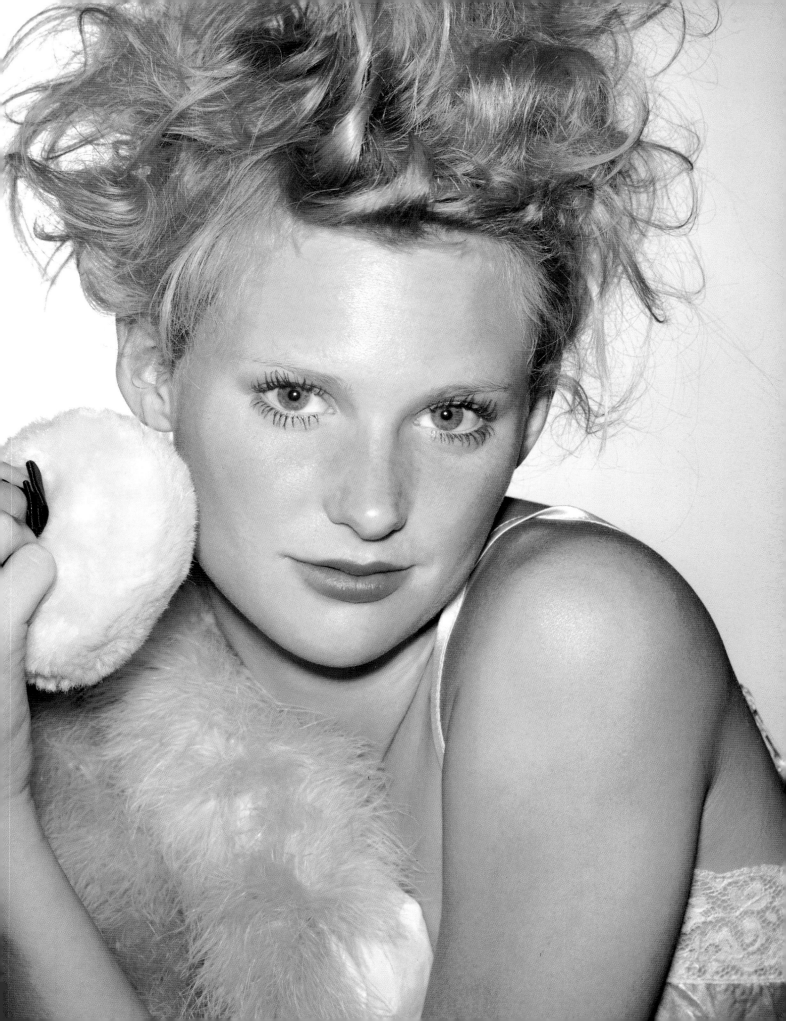

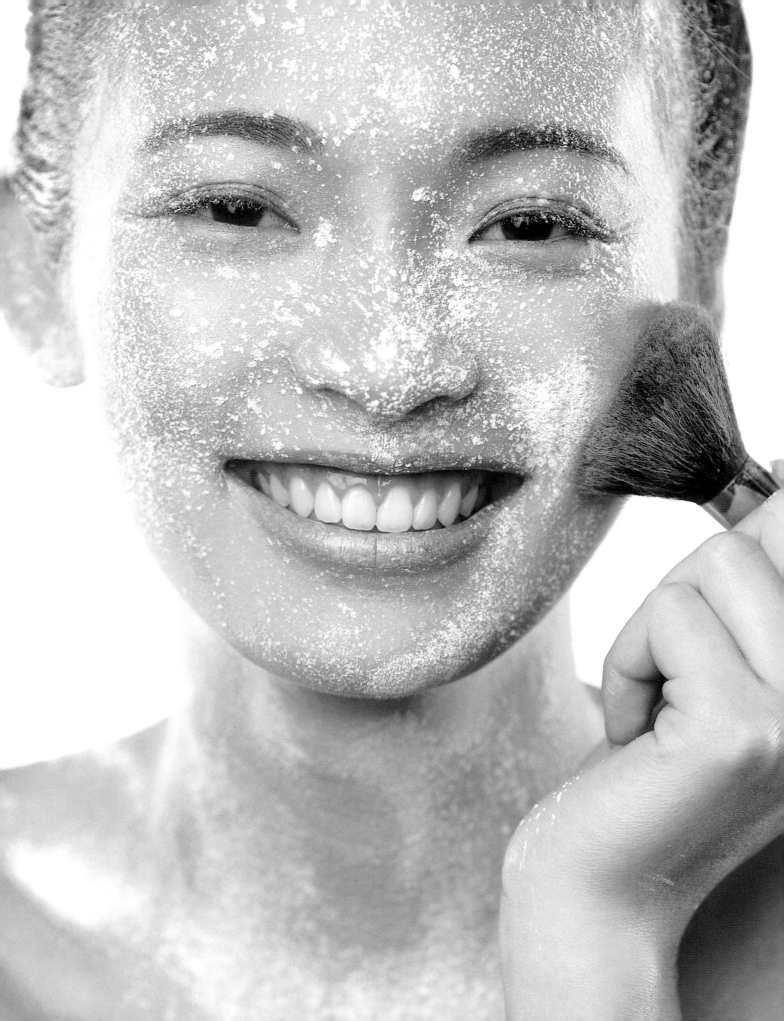

CONCEALERS
& powders

Beautiful, flawless skin is something supermodels are born with, right? Wrong. Pair a few carefully chosen products with the right tools and techniques and make it your birthright too. Ask any make-up artist worth her sable hairbrushes for the best tricks of the trade, and she'll tell you this: "It's not about make-up, it's about skin." If yours is flawless, you can leave your make-up in the drawer and still look stunning; if it's less than perfect – well, a good concealer will help minimize signs of fatigue, age and sun damage, even camouflaging a blemish or two. While powder is the final step in protecting and preserving all your hard work.

CONCEALERS

Concealers have come a long way since the heavy, cloying formulations of the past. Concealer can hide a multitude of flaws, from dark circles under your eyes to blemishes, pigmentation marks, birthmarks and freckles. While faithful lipstick-shaped concealers are still around, we now also have push-up and sponge-tip pens, make-up artist's palettes and mini-tube concealers.

Even if women don't wear any other make-up, most will use it at some time in their lives. For dark circles, lines and the odd spot, nothing beats a concealer. Peachy or slightly yellow-toned concealers are best for under-eye shadows as they help minimize the blue-grey tinge of dark circles. Pink-toned concealers are too cool and will merely emphasize the greyish colour. Newer formulations contain light-reflective pigments that bounce light away from problem areas.

A light concealer on a raised spot is only going to make it stand out more, so it's crucial when concealing raised blemishes to match it exactly to your skin tone or to go for a shade slightly darker to make the skin appear flatter. An oil-free stick concealer is the best all-round option for cover-up work. Steer clear of oil-based preparations as they have a tendency to slide on and then glide off, or to settle into fine lines and wrinkles. Look for a shade that is slightly lighter than your choice of foundation. If you can't find the exact colour match, try mixing a couple of shades on the back of your hand before applying.

Concealer is great for correcting mistakes and disguising all sorts of blemishes:

■ It disguises a badly drawn lip line.

■ It conceals red skin around the nostrils.

■ Applied to eyelids, it offers a great base for eye shadows, helping it to last longer.

■ It lightens and brightens skin eroded from saline tears, taking years off your face.

■ When the lip area seems too dark, apply with a fine brush around the lip line to lighten the area.

■ To counteract red eyes: outline the eyes with a very fine line of concealer, push it into the skin around the eyes right up into the lashes. It 'opens' the eyes and helps to minimize redness.

Choosing colour

Make-up artists suggest testing concealer shades on the inside of your arm. If you're trying to mask blue tones and hide dark circles then go for a concealer with yellow undertones, a few shades lighter than your skin. If you're masking pimples, or evening out skin tone, a yellow undertone is also a good idea – pink shades will only emphasize redness.

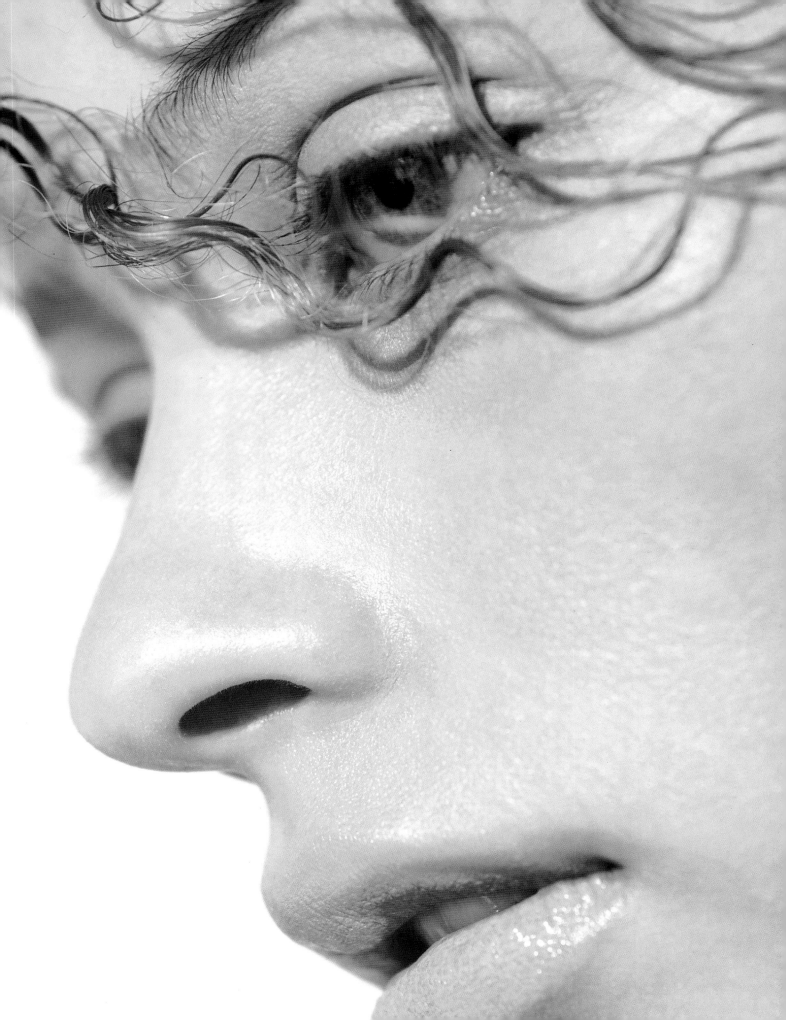

OVER THE TOP

Perhaps the cleverest thing about modern concealer is its ability to work under or over your make-up. If you need a little erasing action, just blend the concealer over your existing make-up. You can apply concealer under foundation and touch up the under-eye area afterwards, but most make-up artists apply foundation first. You'll probably need two kinds of concealer: a fine, light-reflective one for under the eyes and a denser, pigment-rich formula to conceal blemishes.

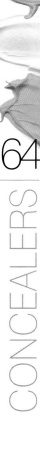

Light-diffusing concealers

Light-diffusing concealers are ideal for lifting the tired points of the face – the corners of the nostrils, eyes and mouth. Their ultra-light texture is also good for those who don't like to wear anything else on their skin. About the only thing you shouldn't do with light-reflective concealers – apart from use them on pimples – is dance under a UV disco light unless you're trying to scare someone. Without blemish ingredients, they can emphasize bumps.

Concealing scars and birthmarks

Scars and birthmarks can be disguised using specially formulated concealers from specialist make-up shops. Concealers developed for television or photographic make-up will offer great coverage and are also available in water-resistant and waterproof formulations to make sure they stay put in all sorts of conditions.

Blemish fighters

If you're covering spots with a concealing stick it is better to find one that contains active ingredients such as tea tree or arnica to heal as it conceals. Many old-style concealers consisted of little more than oil and pigment, which could aggravate the problem.

Primers

If you suffer from high colour or pigmentation problems, spend time priming your skin before applying make-up. To create the perfect canvas for make-up application you need to be meticulous – mistakes here can be disastrous.

Colour correctors

These are coloured liquids or creams that correct skin tones. They counterbalance opposing hues, tone down or brighten the complexion and camouflage imperfections. Use after your moisturizer but before your base, or mixed into your foundation. Apply carefully with a fine-tipped bush, then blend thoroughly with your fingertips.

Green takes redness out of blemishes, thread veins, sunburn and ruddy cheeks; *lilac* revives a tired, sallow complexion; *blue* works well on pale skin; and *apricot* enhances tired skin.

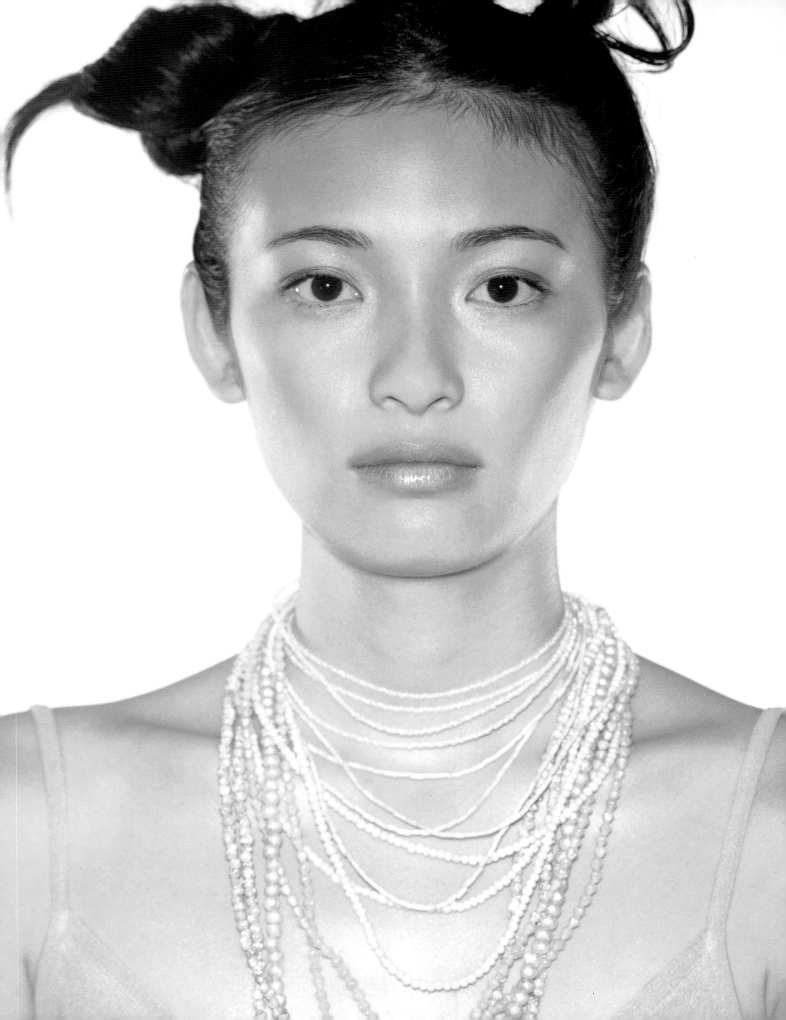

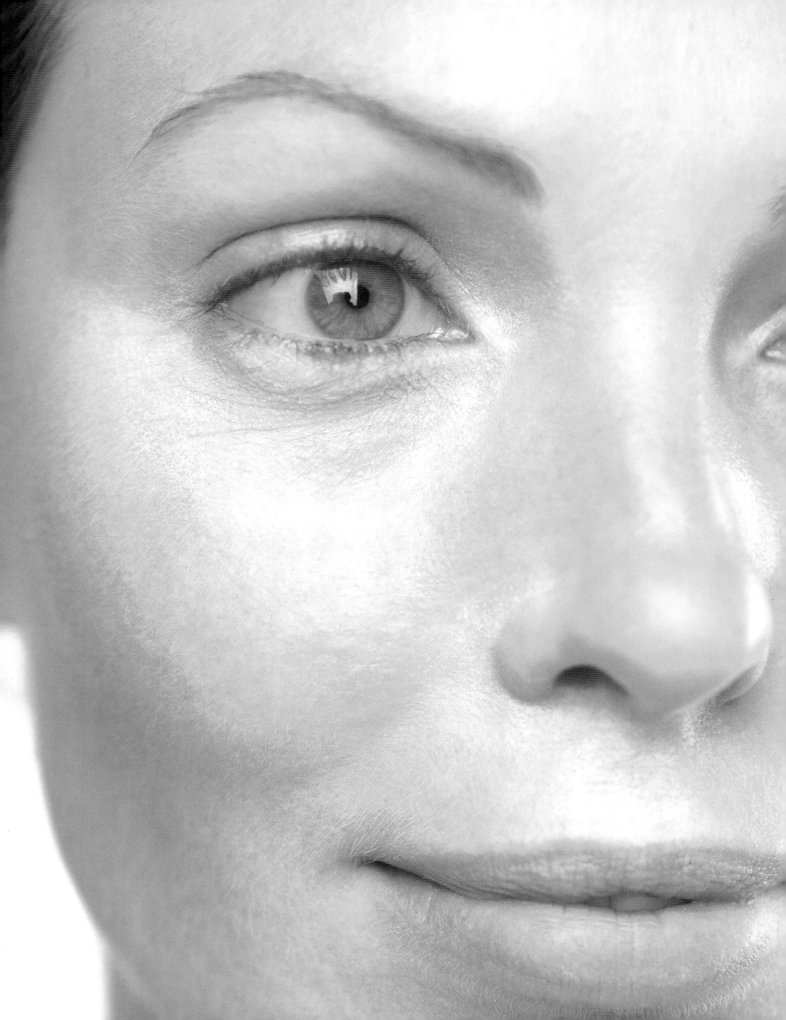

APPLYING CONCEALER

Apply your concealer on top of your foundation and before you add powder. If you try to do things the other way around, you might wipe the concealer off when applying your foundation. Most professional make-up artists tend to do the corrective concealing and highlighting work first, before applying foundation, but that works best once you have become truly proficient.

Tips

- Use a lighter shade to highlight and bring forward, and a darker one to push back and thus conceal an offending area: a light-reflecting one to lift tired areas of the face – the sides of the nostrils and the corners of the mouth and eyes – and one slightly darker than your foundation to minimize bumps.
- Choose a cream, compact or solid stick for covering spots. These formulations are richer in pigment and powder particles and provide intense coverage.
- To mask imperfections, use a fine-tipped make-up brush. Concentrate concealer on the centre of the imperfection and feather outwards. Tap gently to blend and set with powder.
- To prevent contamination in the tube, clean the brush regularly or apply with a cotton bud.
- Choose a formulation that spreads evenly without being too transparent. Use your ring finger to tap the product over the shadow; let it settle to see if more is needed. Better to go quickly and lightly, and then add more, than to apply it too thickly initially.
- To conceal broken capillaries or uneven skin tone, use light brush strokes to apply concealer and then blend with a fingertip.
- To conceal bags under the eyes, apply concealer on the shadow beneath the bag, not on top of the bag itself or you'll highlight rather than disguise the problem.
- To disguise under-eye shadows, gently pat concealer along the orbital bone under the eyes. Exert gentle pressure and blend outwards being careful not to pull or drag the skin.
- Set the area with a fine dusting of powder. For dark circles under the eyes, again apply concealer on the shadow beneath or you will highlight rather than disguise the problem.
- If you don't have your concealer handy, a brush dipped in foundation and layered slightly, will minimize unsightly blemishes and under-eye circles. But bear in mind concealer is more opaque and longer lasting than foundation.
- As signs of ageing become more obvious around the eyes, avoid using powder, as it will emphasize these lines.

CONCEAERS

POWDERS

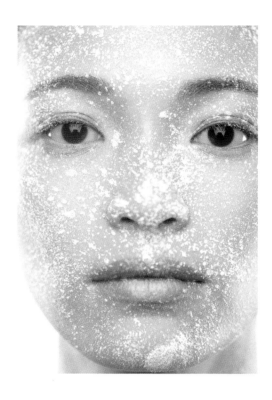

Powder is an important part of applying your foundation, yet women rarely use it other than as a hastily applied dab on a shiny nose. Once considered thick and chalky, new powder formulations are feather light and essential for setting make-up. Powder is the magic wand of make-up. As long as you have it on hand, you can blend away most make-up mistakes and problems. There are two kinds of powder – loose to set your base and pressed or compact to use on its own or for touch-ups during the day. You can use it to:

- make foundation and concealer stay in place, particularly cream-based products that tend to slip and slide
- make lipstick last longer by gently powdering over the first lipstick application
- create a smooth, refined surface that helps colour cosmetics brush on easily and smoothly without blotching and creasing
- unify foundation texture and lighten a too-heavy application of blusher or eye shadow
- keep oily secretions at bay and absorb unwanted moisture, although too much can be ageing.

Choosing powder colour

- Powders come in all shades, but the most effective are translucent or colourless because they can be worn by all skin colours and won't alter or affect the colour of your concealer or foundation.
- If you want the added coverage of a colour powder, keep it neutral and find a shade slightly lighter than your foundation – yellow tones are the most convincing; pink tones are to be avoided at all costs.
- Avoid powders with too much shimmer during the day – you don't want to twinkle. This is especially true if you have dark skin, because shimmery powders can make your skin look grey. Rather choose a yellow or slightly orange-toned powder to match your skin tone.
- If you don't like foundation but hate shiny skin, look for a powder that matches your skin tone exactly and wear it over bare skin. If you have black or dark skin, avoid powders with mica, because they emphasize shiny skin.
- To determine if a powder is good quality, test it on the back of your hand; it should feel silky and smooth and very light. If it looks chalky and heavy, or clogs up in the fine lines on your hand, this means it has not been finely milled and will show up on your face.

Application tips

■ Leave your foundation to settle for a few minutes before dusting on powder.

■ Dip your brush into the powder, gently blow any excess off the bristles. Work down the face to prevent particles of powder from catching superfluous facial hair and giving an uneven finish. Sweep to blend.

■ If you're going to apply eye make-up, dab a fairly thick coating of translucent powder under the crescent area of your eye area beforehand to collect any deposits of eye shadow that fall down. The powder will act as a magnet for any falling eye shadow. Sweep away with a soft brush when you have fin-ished blending to avoid leaving your face streaked with colour. (This tip is not recommended for older skins.)

■ If using a velour puff for application, lightly press on face and roll, repeating motion to literally press powder into the skin. This cre-ates a longer-lasting finish and is better for oily skin types.

■ A powder brush is domed and won't cover all areas, but because it skims the surface, it's useful for sweep-ing away excess powder. Generally, the more soft and voluminous the brush and the more natural the fibre, the better.

■ Gently place a little powder under the eyes, down the bridge of your nose and onto the tip of your chin.

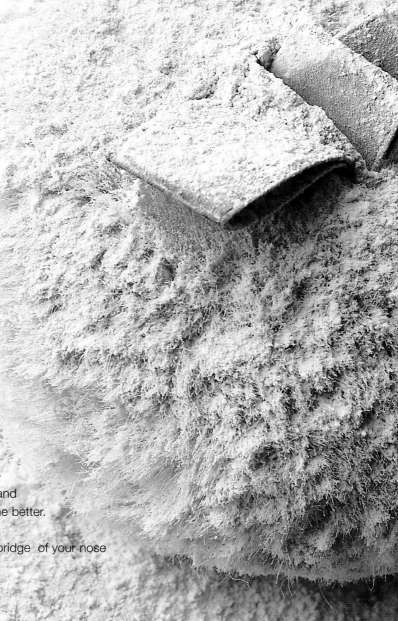

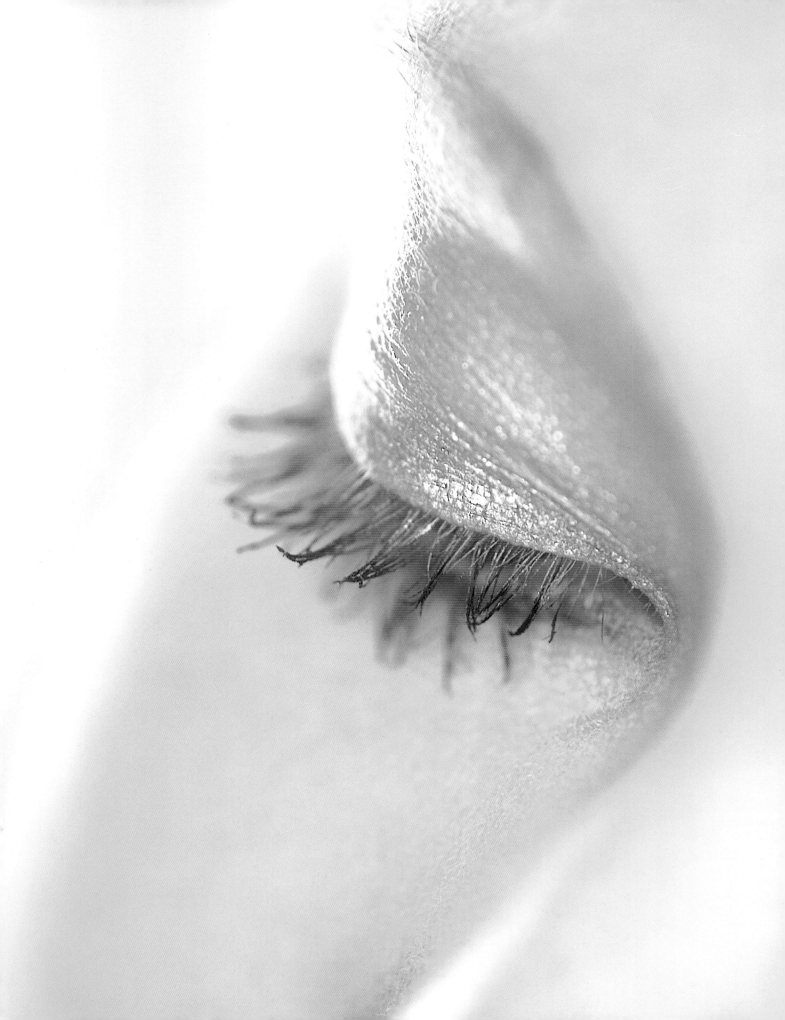

Eye shadow can shimmer subtly or gleam dramatically. It can also be maddeningly hard to master, which is probably why so many women don't bother. If it's true that eyes are the windows to the soul, eye shadow is the window dressing. It can be as simple as a neutral sweep on the lid or as involved as multicolour, shadow play from eyelid to eyebrow. Aside from some general rules – like not wearing anything that's too dark and glitzy for daywear, or clown colours – the hardest part is choosing from a huge array of options. Fashion trends help narrow the choices, but if you're like me you shouldn't follow the pack: experiment until you find what suits you and look to trends for inspiration.

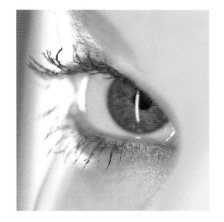

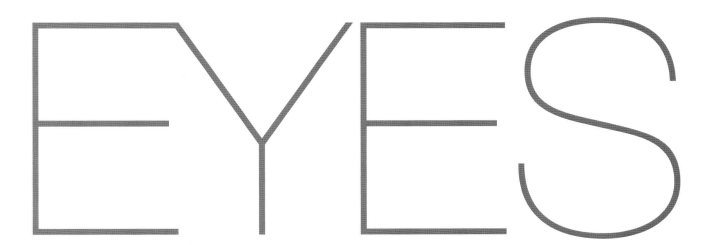

"Don't follow the pack: experiment until you find the look that suits you."

TIRED EYE RESCUE

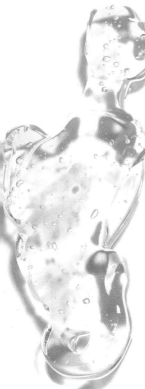

Quick fixes. A soothing slick of ice or a teaspoon cooled in icy water applied around the eyes do wonders to perk up slack, tired skin. Or try courgette or cucumber slices soaked in cooled ginseng tea.

For dark circles. Use an eye cream or gel that is formulated to reduce dark circles – an anti-ageing, anti-wrinkle eye cream won't necessarily do the job.

For puffy eyes. Deflate bags with a cooling astringent gel. Splashing your face with cold water also helps reduce bags under the eyes. Don't apply concealer, as it will just accentuate the bags. Instead, brush a little translucent powder under the eyes to prevent excess shine and reduce the appearance of bags – a reflective surface attracts light and tends to look bigger.

Ban the oil. Don't remove your eye make-up with baby oil. Anything laden with oils can seep into your eyes, cause puffiness and irritate tear ducts.

Eye cream application. The skin around the eye area is thin and tends to be drier as there are fewer oil glands there. Applying eye cream too close to your eyes can cause puffiness. Rather dab gently onto the orbital bone with your ring finger every morning and night.

Sleep. Nothing can replace eight solid hours of shut-eye. Night-time is the ultimate time for repair.

Eye openers

Quick fixes. To instantly 'open' and brighten up dull eyes, use a white pencil to line the lower inner rim of your eyelids.

To camouflage dark circles. Try a moisturizing gel with optical diffusers that won't congeal or build up under the eyes – one that won't let your concealer slide off. Matte concealers are best, and the colour needs to be light enough to cover the dark circles but not too light. Yellow or slightly orange undertones help to counteract the bluish tinge of under-eye circles. Tilt your head down, then look up into a mirror – your black rings will look very obvious but you will see precisely where to apply concealer. Most people apply concealer under the entire eye area, but it's unnecessary and it can give you panda eyes. Apply just where the hollow appears. Avoid waxy pencils along the lower lashes; rather opt for a powder to line the lower lashes.

Brow lift. Neat brows do wonders to perk up your face. If you need extra definition, use an eye shadow powder to enhance them. If you must pluck, remove only those straggly hairs growing beneath the brow. If your 'arch' is missing, recreate one by using a soft, natural shade of brow pencil along the upper edge of the brow to give you 'lift'.

Fake it. By adding a few individual false eyelashes to the outer corner of your eyes to extend your lash line, you'll be creating a wide-eyed doe effect. If that sounds like too much bother, add an outward sweep of liquid eyeliner on the outer corner for added oomph.

Curl it. Lash curlers are renowned for their eye-opening abilities. Always curl lashes before applying mascara. Keep lash curlers clean and the rubber lining in good condition to prevent sharp edges from snipping off your lashes.

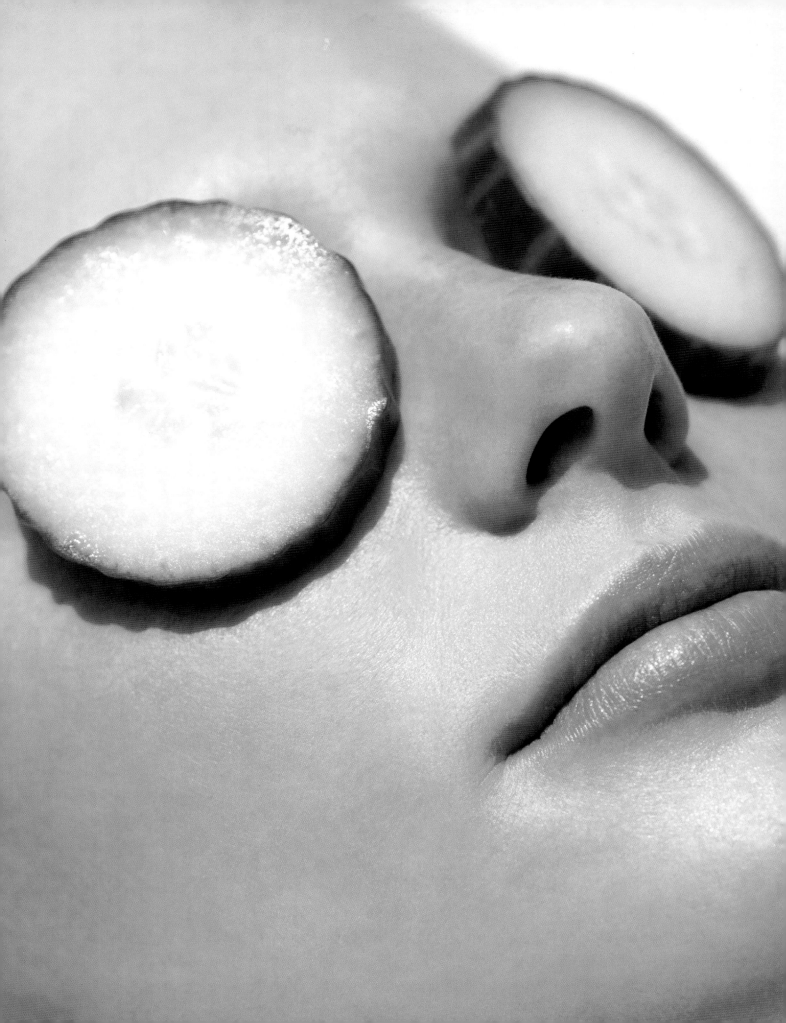

EYEBROWS

Perfectly groomed eyebrows can frame your face, brighten your eyes, and make you look younger. If they aren't groomed, nothing else you do looks quite right. To get your brows in their best shape can be difficult. Here are some pointers:

Assemble your tools. You'll need a sharp set of tweezers with tips that meet, a clean eyebrow brush, a white or light-coloured eye pencil and a well-lit mirror. If you're worried about plucking pain, massage with an ice cube to numb the area or dab on a bit of anaesthetic cream with a cotton bud. Some make-up artists keep a tube of teething gel for this purpose.

Determine your shape. The most important element of shapely brows is a well-placed arch. The highest part of your arch should be above the outer edge of your iris.

Map out your moves. Brush your eyebrows straight up and use a white eye pencil to draw on the line of your arch from the point closest to your nose out toward your temple. You'll pluck the hairs that fall under the line to give you the most natural look.

Go slow. You don't want to end up taking out too many hairs. Hold your skin taut and pluck one hair at a time in the direction of the hair growth. Stop once you've plucked all the hairs under the white line.

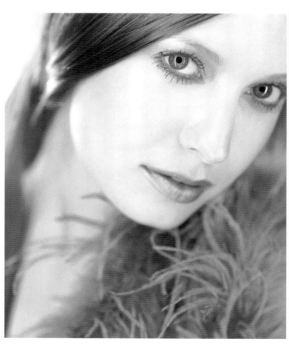
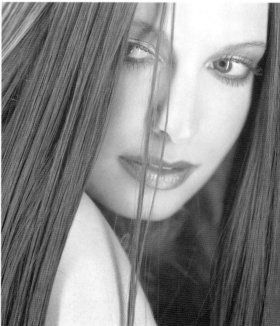

Essential tools

- The first step to perfect brows: perfect tweezers. Look for a pair with sharp, slanted tips, which allow you to pluck even the shortest, finest hairs.

- Set unruly eyebrows with a clear brow gel. Its mascara-like wand distributes the gel evenly, so you get all-over hold.

- An eyebrow pencil in a shade lighter than your hair colouring. Apply using short, upward strokes to mimic the hair growth, rather than a solid line, to create a softer, natural effect.

- Shapeless, fair brows can be emphasized by applying powder in a shade lighter than your hair, unless your hair is very blonde. Apply colour in short strokes, following the brow bone for a natural finish.

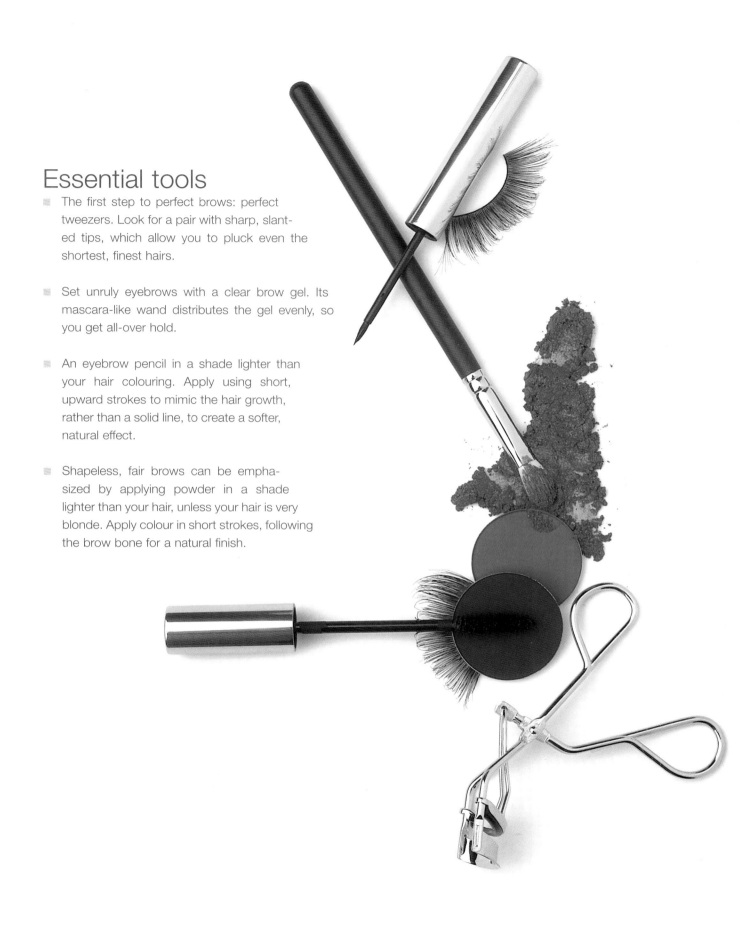

EYEBROW TIPS

Ten common brow mistakes
- Not plucking at all
- Over-thinning ends
- Not taming unruly brows
- Not filling in sparse brows
- Plucking too much under the arch
- Plucking too much between brows
- Creating a shape that doesn't look natural
- Creating the 'tadpole' shape, which makes your eyes look close-set
- Forming bald patches because you pluck from within the body of the eyebrow

- Use a warm, damp face cloth to open pores so that tweezing is easier and less painful. The best time to pluck your eyebrows is after a bath or shower. Remember to pluck in the direction of the hair growth.
- For the most natural look don't reshape above your natural brow line; only pluck stray hairs or bleach unwanted growth with carefully applied facial hair lightener.
- Do not make your eyebrows too short. Use the pencil test: hold a pencil flat along the side of your nose. This is where your eyebrow should begin. Then pivot the pencil, keeping the end next to your nostril, to the outer corner of your eye. This is where your eyebrow should stop.
- Tweeze one row of hairs at a time on alternate brows to ensure an even match. It can take eight weeks for them to grow back. Be warned: overplucking can lead to permanent loss.
- Try not to over- or underarch your brows. The ideal geometry is: lowest at the inner ends, close to the nose; highest at the top of the arch; and tapered at the far ends to form a triangle or arch. Better yet, have them professionally shaped, then pluck to maintain the shape.
- Don't pluck from within the body of the eyebrow because you'll end up with gaps. Trim rogue stragglers with nail scissors.
- Fill in sparse areas with eye pencil or matching matte eye shadow. Your choice of pencil should depend on the colour of your brows – opt for a shade lighter.
- While bleaching or dyeing the brows to match your hair colour is vital to pulling off a natural-looking hairstyle, eyebrow pencils are another, easier, more convenient method.
- Remember, the more you pluck away from beneath your brows, the greater the space you create for applying eye make-up.

How to flatter your face shape

- To soften a squarish face, arch brows above the pupils.
- If your face is oval, slant brows upwards slightly at the ends to open eyes.
- Keep brows horizontal to draw attention from a long rectangular face.
- Round face shapes should keep brows neat, short and upswept.

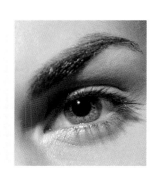

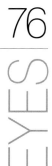

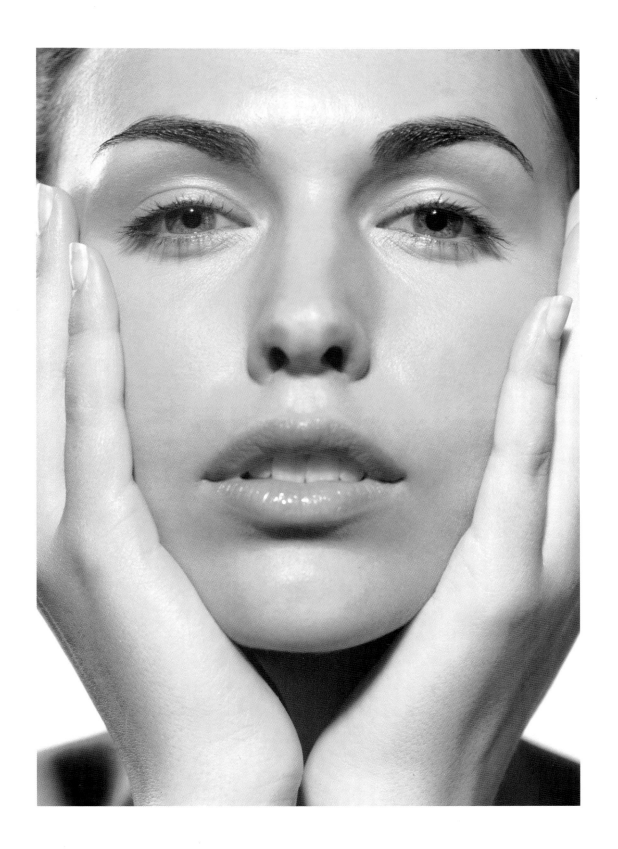

EYE-SHADOW FORMULATIONS

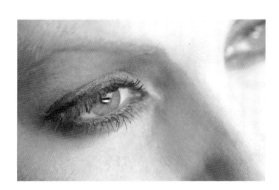

Shadows are available in matte or shimmer finishes. Matte finishes offer a more natural look, are safer and easier to work with. Beware of shimmery and frosted textures if you have mature lids; they accentuate the skin's texture.

Powders and cream powders are popular and easy to control. The powders are applied with a brush and cover large areas. Cream powders usually come in squeezable tubes or bottles with sponge-tip applicators. On application they dry to a powder finish.

Pencils offer concentrated colour and can double as eyeliner. Some come with sponge-tip applicators and help with blending.

Creams come in pots and wand-style applicators. Fairly easy to apply, they do however, leave crease marks and fade easily. Set with powder to make them last.

Choosing colour

Experimentation is the way to find out what works for you, but for a basic face, nothing beats neutral shades. Everything from vanilla to almond, to mid-tones like taupe and terracotta, to deep shades like coffee and smoky grey. Ultimately your own colouring will determine what works best for you. Redheads, for instance, look great with peachy, orange shades, while black skins work brilliantly with mochas and deep burgundies. The basic rules: pale green or violet for skins with yellow undertones; use pale blue sparingly or it'll look harsh; and keep lip and cheek colours neutral when wearing stronger eye shadows. But one tip: single eye shadows are usually the better buy – you'll seldom use all the shades in a trio compact.

Anti-ageing

Eyes seem to present the biggest challenge as we age: make-up just doesn't seem to work the way it used to, mainly because it settles into fine lines and wrinkles. To apply make-up to older eyes, open the eye area by gently holding the eyebrow up. This allows you to apply shadow all over the lid, rather than just the area that's visible.

Keep to a fairly neutral palette and leave funky colours to teenagers, as bright colours can be very ageing. Stick to smoky-grey, brown and pink-toned blushers. Also forget that old-fashioned idea of matching your eye shadows to your eyes. If you have brown eyes, try emphasizing them with grey shades; if your eyes are blue or grey, go for browns.

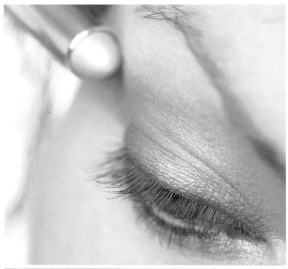

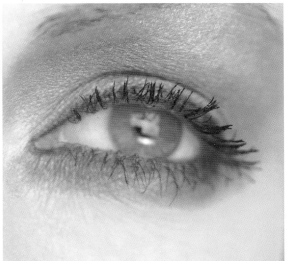

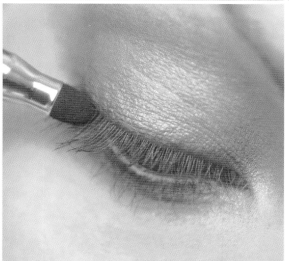

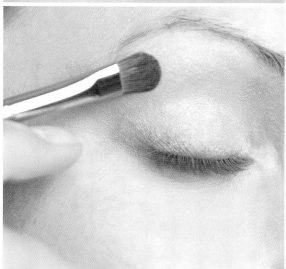

Anti-ageing tips

- Avoid frosted iridescent shadows containing mica, a pearlized powder, which settles into and emphasizes fine lines and wrinkles.

- Look for long-lasting matte shades of eye shadow. Matte and lighter shades lift and open the eye area, while shiny, iridescent eye shadows, even if in fashion, emphasize crepe-like skin.

- The silly sponge applicators that come with most eye shadow compacts should be thrown away. Not only are they very fiddly, but they drag the skin, which may contribute to further lines and wrinkles. Brushes are gentler on the delicate eye area.

- Avoid liquid eyeliner, which becomes increasingly more difficult to apply as the crêpe-like character of the skin increases with age. Rather opt for a pencil or a powder shadow applied with a blunt brush, which is softer and more flattering.

- Deep-set eyes need bringing out – apply a pale colour across the entire upper lid from the lash line to the brow.

EYES MADE UP

Prime your canvas. An artist doesn't just start slathering paint onto fresh canvas, just as a make-up artist doesn't work on a surface that hasn't been prepared. Prime the area with a light concealer or foundation and a dusting of translucent powder to control oiliness and help set the colour. Although priming is always a good idea, it's absolutely non-negotiable if you're using a cream-formula shadow. Avoid using a heavy textured concealer on the eyelid – it tends to gunk up shadow.

Apply a base shade. Pick a light, a dark, and a medium shade. It's easier if they're in the same colour family – like bone, taupe, and dark brown – but they don't have to be. And bear in mind, if you're using multiple colours, powdered shadow is much easier to control because it layers and blends easily. It's possible to combine cream and powder, but not cream and cream – they'll mush together. The lightest shade opens up the eye area – dust on the entire lid, from the brow to the lash line.

Shade for contrast. The medium shade is the one that's going to bring out the colour of your eyes, so look for a suitably contrasting shade. Green eyes will stand out when shaded with browns and a hint of red; blue eyes are complemented by purple shades. And brown eyes work with any colour, as long as it's not an exact match – the shadow should be darker or paler than the eye itself. Or try a neutral shade like grey, brown or off-white. Apply this second shade across the lid to a point just above the crease and then blend lightly.

Three ways to wear eye shadow

1 **A wash of colour on entire lid.** The easiest of all shadow techniques, simply use a large eye-shadow brush, and starting at the lash line blend powder to just over the crease, blending upwards and outwards. To widen eyes use a light colour; to minimize them use a medium shade.

2 **A medium shade worn in the crease.** This creates depth, which brings the eyes forward. Using a medium-sized brush, follow the natural contour of the lid. The shadow should extend a little above the crease so that you can see it when your eyes are open. Colour can be intensified in the corners for extra definition, but don't take it beyond the corners.

3 **A dark colour worn next to lash line.** This creates definition. With a pencil or a fine eye-shadow brush, place a smudged line near the top, the bottom, or on both lash lines. This emphasizes the eyes and makes lashes look fuller. The line should be thicker at the outer corners and fade towards the inner eyes.

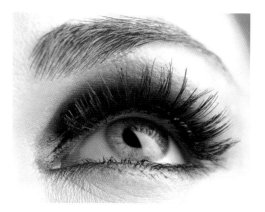

Line the lashes. Take the darkest shade and a small brush. An angled brush with hard bristles is easiest to manoeuvre. Dampen the brush and dunk it into a little powder, then make a slightly smudgy line around the lashes – either top and bottom or top only. When dark colour is applied only below the eye, it draws attention to eye bags and makes you look tired. The important thing is to get as close to the lash line as possible. When you've finished, use a large, fluffy brush to sweep away any stray shadow that has fallen onto the cheek.

Tips

- If the eye make-up you're planning is complicated, do your foundation afterwards. That way you don't have to worry about stray flecks of glitter ruining your foundation.

- When working with a few colours, always start with the lightest shades first.

- Before applying shadow, always give the brush a little flick, or blow gently to remove excess powder.

- Blend well; you should never be able to tell where one colour begins and ends.

- Dark shadows make an area recede, light ones make an area come forward.

- Use a highlighter on any part of the eye area that you want to bring out. Put a dot on the inner corner of the eye to make eyes look big and bright, and a dab under the arch of the brow to emphasize the brows, if necessary.

- Don't over-emphasize the brow bone; most times the absence of colour is enough of a highlight. I see many make-up artists using very pearlized or white shadows as a highlighter and it really creates an artificial effect best avoided.

- Don't use dark colours in the corner of your eyelids nearest your nose; this will pull the eyes in, and make even the smallest nose look larger.

- If your eyes are close-set, concentrate colour on the centre of the eye moving outwards, and avoid the inner corner. This will create the illusion of wide-set eyes.

- If your eyes are deep-set, avoid dark colours in the crease of the eyes; it creates bug-eyes.

- Cream or powder? Powder is the better option if you're a control freak. Some women in tropical climates prefer cream powder, essentially because it's so sheer and easy to apply with the fingers, but it tends to slip and slide on the lid, accumulating in the crease line and requiring touch-ups. (Dusting with translucent powder underneath and over the cream helps.) Ultimately powder is easier to blend, more stable and allows you to build up layers for a more intense saturated colour.

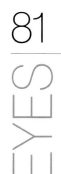

LASHES

Eyeliner

Liner helps define shape and opens the eye, but it should be done with a delicate line. Black liner is only for those with dark hair and dark skin, otherwise dark brown is deep enough. Soft brown, taupe and grey tones suit fair skins. Eyeliner pencils give a softer finish than liquids, but the most effective is a dark powder shadow line, which you create by using a tiny, pointed brush.

Liquid liners give a sharp line; they can be difficult to apply and even harder to remove if you make a mistake. It's best left to the professionals, but if you must, here's how. Look down, and with one finger holding the eyelid taut, draw a fine line along the upper lid in one continuous movement as close to the lashes as possible; end at the outer corner, do not extend.

Most women should use liner on the upper lid only – just dot or feather strokes, or a softly smudged line on the bottom if you have no definition there at all. Eyeliner looks better when smudged a little to blend in with lashes and shadow. Pencil is more subtle, less severe and much easier to apply.

Eyelashes

Lashes need to be obvious, not spiky or thick, but long and feathery. Brush and lightly powder lashes to provide a built-up surface for the mascara. It's often an idea to curl them for a more fluttery look. Build up mascara in layers, many thin coats are better than a heavy one.

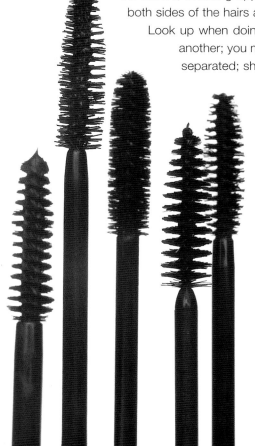

Look down when doing the upper lashes. Start by applying to the tips by sweeping the mascara brush across the lashes, inner corner outwards, almost against the direction of growth. Then wiggle the brush down to the base of the lashes, brushing upper lashes downward from the top, and lower lashes upward from below. This ensures both sides of the hairs are coated, and sweeps the lashes upward.

Look up when doing the lower lashes; brush up first, then down. Allow each layer to dry before applying another; you may need several coats depending on the fullness you want. It's important to keep lashes separated; should they cake and stick together, separate them with a fine, clean eyelash comb.

Eyelash curlers look pretty daunting, but with a little practice you'll be amazed at the results. Curling the lashes opens the eyes, making them look bigger. Place the curler at the base of the lashes (see page 106); squeeze a few times as you work out towards the edge of the lashes.

False eyelashes

False lashes can enhance the loveliest eyes, but they're best left to the pros. Full eyelashes can leave you looking like a drag queen, but single lashes can create a natural effect. Select smaller ones for the inside of the eye, and longer ones for the middle.

Start from the inside and build outwards. With tweezers pick up a lash, dip the base in eyelash glue, press the false lash base against the natural lash base, and hold for a second. To conceal eyelash glue, apply a smoky line of colour along the base of the lash line, and remember to curl the false ones as well as your real set.

Mascara tips

- Avoid the tendency to pump the wand up and down for an even coverage of mascara. This action traps air inside the tube causing the mascara to dry out quickly.

- Use a clear mascara for a natural, slightly dewy look, which is great with minimal make-up. It also doubles up as a styler for shaping brows.

- Place a tissue directly under the lashes when applying mascara to prevent any mess – ideal for nervous and watery eyes.

- If your lashes are quite short, lengthening mascara can make all the difference. Microscopic fibres attach themselves to the end of your lashes, and create the illusion of a lengthy pair of lashes. Avoid the use of lengthening mascara if your eyes are sensitive, though.

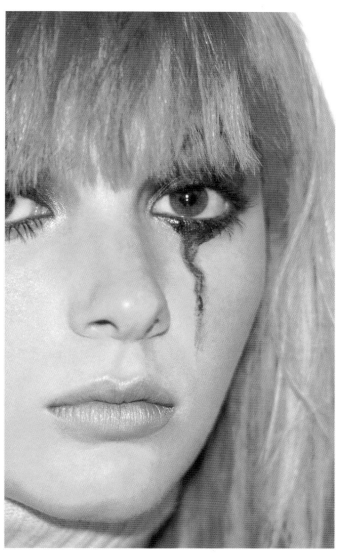

- Thickening mascaras contain silicones that pump up the appearance of your natural set and create the illusion of generous fringing.

- To remove a smudge, dip a cotton bud into a non-oily eye make-up remover and gently rub off unwanted mascara, or dip into foundation and gently wipe away smudge.

- To prevent a mascara wand from becoming too clogged, wash through with soapy water, rinse and leave to dry completely before using.

- If the lashes become stuck together or you can see a clump of mascara, brush through with an eyelash comb or an old, cleaned mascara wand.

- Don't share your mascara with anyone and throw it away after three months.

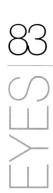

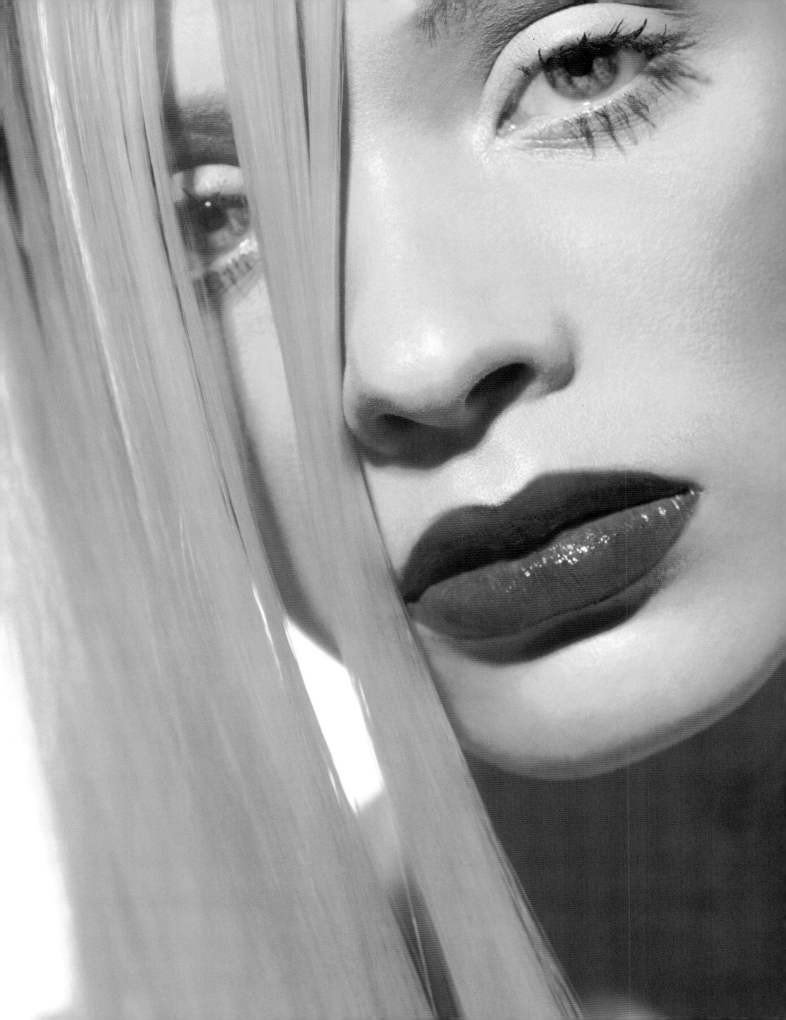

Lipstick is the make-up item most women can least live without. Six out of ten of us apply an extra coat before we answer the doorbell, and we recognize lipstick as the easiest way to update our image – in the same way that changing a hemline can update our wardrobe. It is also the one make-up product that women are most likely to be critical of if, once bought, they dislike its consistency and weight. This is probably because the lips, with their millions of nerve endings, are extremely sensitive. Because there are so many colours to choose from, it's hard to go wrong with lipstick. One day you might want a pale Bardot look and the next, a vampy red Monroe. Nor do you have to stick to one shade. Feel free to mix and match your shades, instantly creating something new.

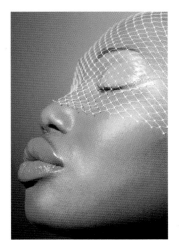

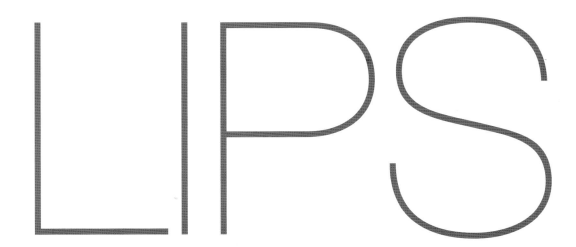

"For some, achieving perfect skin seems impossible, but good skin is achievable. It simply takes work! With a bit of knowledge, your skin will look better – and be healthier – than you ever thought possible ..."

LIP CARE

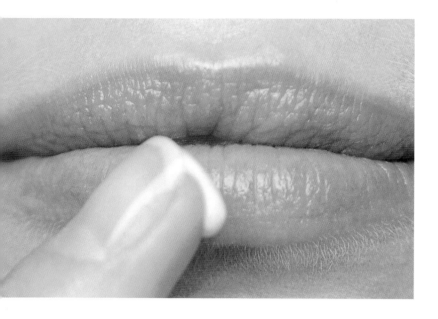

No lipstick is going to look luxurious if lips aren't well cared for first. Since the lips have few oil glands and no ability to create sun-filtering, natural melanin, they provide virtually no protection of their own. Chapped lips are common in winter, when the cold, dry air dehydrates the skin, but bombardment by dry air conditioning, sun and wind, is sure to dry out lips all year round.

Regular use of lip balms offers the fastest remedy for chapped, dry lips. Composed of waxes and oil, some formulas also contain menthol or camphor to soothe rawness and stinging. Others feature allantoin or aloe to speed healing. Many incorporate sunscreen, a must for outdoor exposure, but make sure they contain UVA-protecting ingredients like avobenzone, titanium dioxide, or zinc oxide.

Problems

No lipstick, no matter how creamy, looks good on cracked lips. Preventative care will keep your lips in good shape and condition.

Chapping. To prevent and treat, apply balm daily so that it slightly overlaps the edges of the lips. Look for a balm with sun protection; vitamins A, C or E; and AHAs.

Splitting. Cracks often occur after sleeping in dry air. To prevent this, be sure to apply balm before going to bed, and use a humidifier.

Lipstick bleeding. This begins as the skin around the mouth loses collagen and elastic tissue with age, or is aggravated by smoking. Using a waxy lipliner to outline lips will help contain your lipstick within the line. When cosmetics no longer help, the more permanent (and pricey) solution is to have collagen injections to fill cracks.

Cold sores. Caused by viral infections, these look like blisters or open scabs. To avoid reinfection, use cotton swabs to apply lipstick while sore is visible.

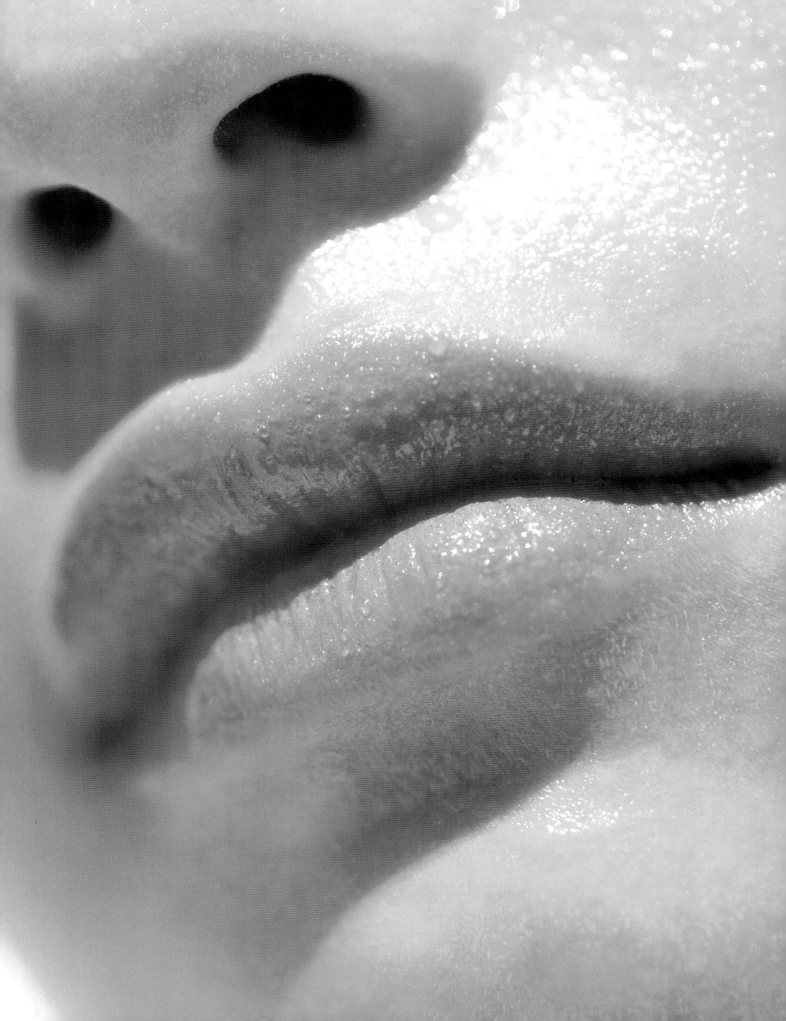

STICK TALK

Transfer-resistant. Lasts up to eight hours but can feel dry on lips.

Long-wearing. Stays put but can feel dry. Look for ingredients like vitamin E, aloe, and ceramides.

Frosted. Shimmery and iridescent due to the light-reflecting mica.

Matte. Colour-rich but moisture-poor. Contains powders that make the pigments opaque and flat.

Cream. Contains lighter waxes, like beeswax or candelilla, which don't dry lips but won't last very long.

Moisturizing. Smooth and shiny, it usually contains vitamin E, aloe or ceramides, but it doesn't last.

Satin/sheer. Glossy and moisturizing due to high oil content but requires frequent reapplication. Looks darker in the tube than on the mouth.

Lip gloss. Applied over lip pencil or dotted on the centre of the lips to create a subtle shine and illusion of fullness. Lip gloss colours are usually transparent and very subtle, but there are some highly pigmented versions available that give lips a wet shiny finish. The only problem with lip gloss is that you need to constantly reapply as it tends to disappear fairly quickly.

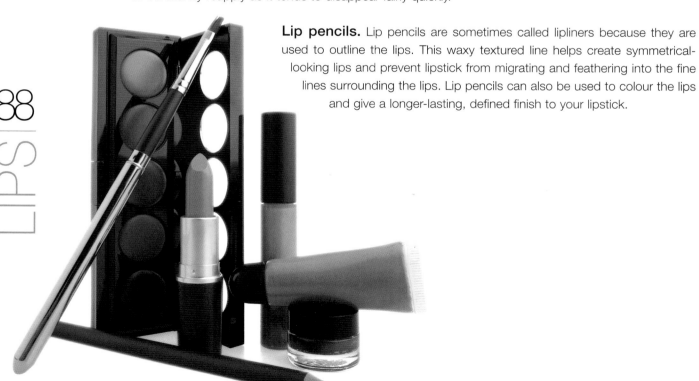

Lip pencils. Lip pencils are sometimes called lipliners because they are used to outline the lips. This waxy textured line helps create symmetrical-looking lips and prevent lipstick from migrating and feathering into the fine lines surrounding the lips. Lip pencils can also be used to colour the lips and give a longer-lasting, defined finish to your lipstick.

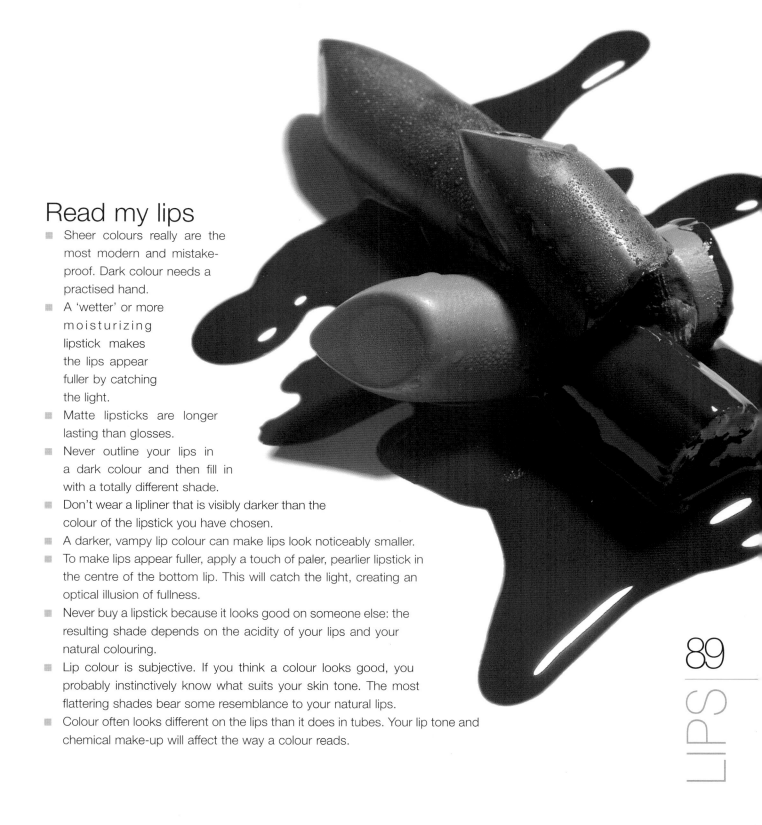

Read my lips

- Sheer colours really are the most modern and mistake-proof. Dark colour needs a practised hand.
- A 'wetter' or more moisturizing lipstick makes the lips appear fuller by catching the light.
- Matte lipsticks are longer lasting than glosses.
- Never outline your lips in a dark colour and then fill in with a totally different shade.
- Don't wear a lipliner that is visibly darker than the colour of the lipstick you have chosen.
- A darker, vampy lip colour can make lips look noticeably smaller.
- To make lips appear fuller, apply a touch of paler, pearlier lipstick in the centre of the bottom lip. This will catch the light, creating an optical illusion of fullness.
- Never buy a lipstick because it looks good on someone else: the resulting shade depends on the acidity of your lips and your natural colouring.
- Lip colour is subjective. If you think a colour looks good, you probably instinctively know what suits your skin tone. The most flattering shades bear some resemblance to your natural lips.
- Colour often looks different on the lips than it does in tubes. Your lip tone and chemical make-up will affect the way a colour reads.

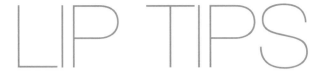

LIP TIPS

Lips need shine, colour, and careful shaping. Learn to outline lips, using a pencil or brush and a tone that is darker or lighter than the overall colour. This gives a cleaner, neater, fresher look than stick colour alone. For greater control, rest your elbow on a table using your hand as a lever. Outline bottom lip first, from centre to right corner, from centre to left corner. Fill in with colour either with a brush or the lipstick. Correcting lips is not always successful; alterations can be very obvious, especially when lipstick starts to wear off. Here are a few corrective pointers:

Too big. Outline just inside the natural line using a natural shade, even if your chosen lip colour is different. A neutral shade will look more natural. Fill in with a deeper matte colour, which absorbs light instead of reflecting it, helping the mouth to appear smaller. Detract attention from the mouth by filling in the new lip shape with a neutral liner, and creating dramatic eyes, instead.

Too full. Avoid bright, shiny or intense colours. Keep lipstick inside natural lip line; outline in matching shade. If you make a mistake, remove the line with cleanser on a cotton bud, and apply concealer to the exposed area before starting again.

Too thin. Using a slightly blunt lipliner, trace just outside the natural lipline, following its natural shape and stopping a little short at the corners. Fill in with a deeper tone. Apply a touch of gold or silver as a highlighter to the centre of the bottom lip for added fullness. Light, glossy colours create the appearance of fuller lips; avoid anything too dark or too matte.

Uneven colour. Balance different-coloured lips by covering both with a little foundation. Outline lips with a lipliner, then brush in a darker shade on the lip that looks lighter and a lighter shade on the one that looks darker. Purse the lips gently together to even out the colour further.

Ageing lips. As we age the skin barrier function becomes less efficient, meaning that moisture escapes more easily. Over time lips get thinner and paler in colour. Lipliner is absolutely essential for mature skin; it creates a waxy barrier that holds lipstick in place and prevents it from feathering and bleeding over the edges. Find a shade that matches your natural lip tone and fill in the entire lip for longer lasting lipstick.

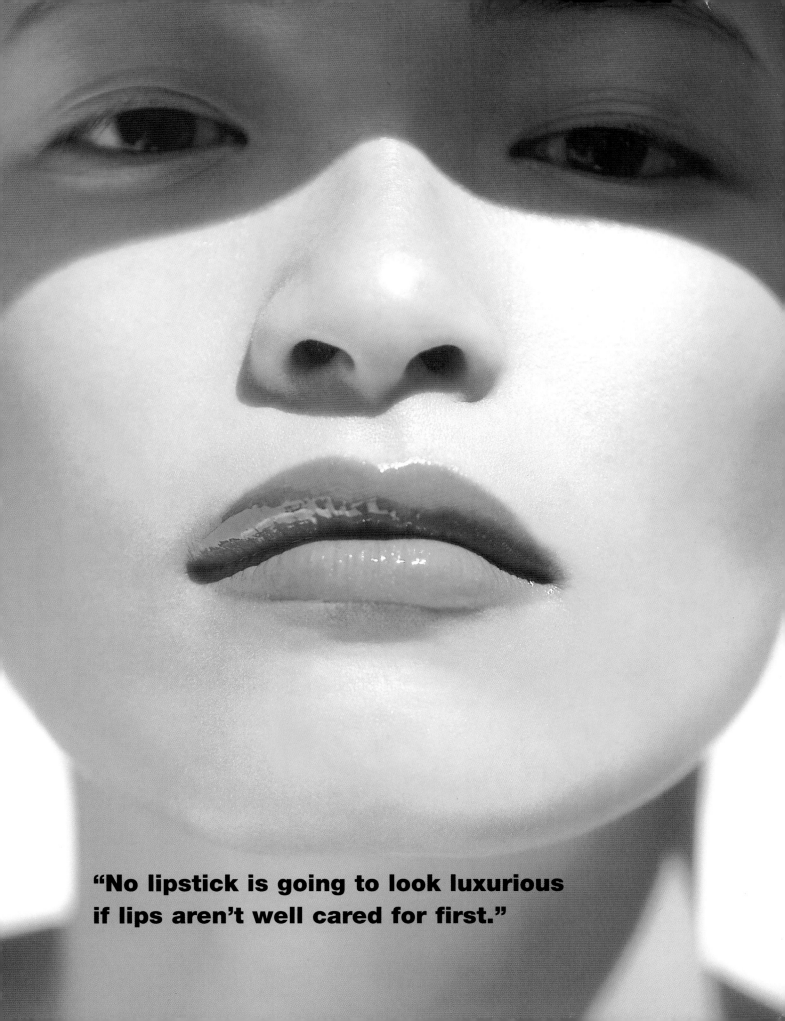

"No lipstick is going to look luxurious
if lips aren't well cared for first."

APPLICATION TIPS

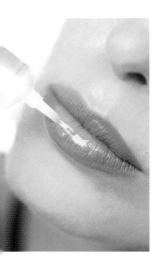

Lips tend to dry out because they have no sebaceous glands. Take a toothbrush and brush Vaseline or lip balm into them. This will help exfoliate any dead skin, seal in moisture and act as a primer for lipstick. The waxiness works to fill cracks and smooth the lip surface.

- Since lips contain no melanin, they need protection against the sun's burning rays. So when you're out in the sun, protect lips with a screen that has a high SPF.

- Always use a brush when applying lipstick for a precise look. The brush allows you to get right into the corners without smudging and it ensures that you keep your colour within your lipline rather than smudging it over the edges.

- To achieve a soft, tidy line and prevent bleeding without lining lips, try soaking a cotton bud in liquid foundation, or concealer, and run it around the outside of an already-painted mouth.

- When using a lip pencil sharpen it before use. This not only ensures a precise point but also takes away any greasy residual on the pencil tip and reveals the fresh crayon underneath, making application much easier. Avoid making it too sharp or it will create a harsh outline. Use it lightly to trace the outer edges of your lips, keeping your lips relaxed to avoid creating unnatural shapes.

- After outlining your lips with a pencil, use it to colour in your lips, even if you're applying lipstick on top. This allows colour to wear off uniformly so that you aren't left with a hard outline after eating.

- In a hurry? Rub colour into your lips using your middle finger to create a stain. A slightly uneven edge looks more natural. Forget about lipliner.

- To keep lipstick off teeth, apply colour with a brush and then blot. Hold a finger horizontally between lips and bite down, pulling your finger out to remove any lipstick that could rub off on your teeth.

- Blot your lipstick with a tissue and then reapply to build up colour and durability.

- Use a brush to get to the bottom of your lipstick – there are often 20 more applications at the base.

- Remember, any kind of oil will dissolve lipstick on contact, including salad dressing!

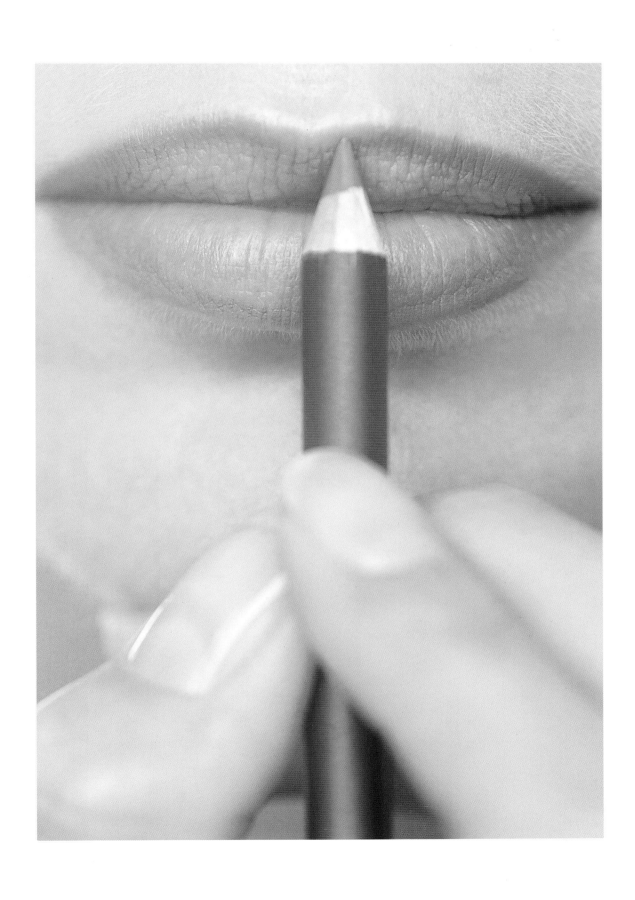

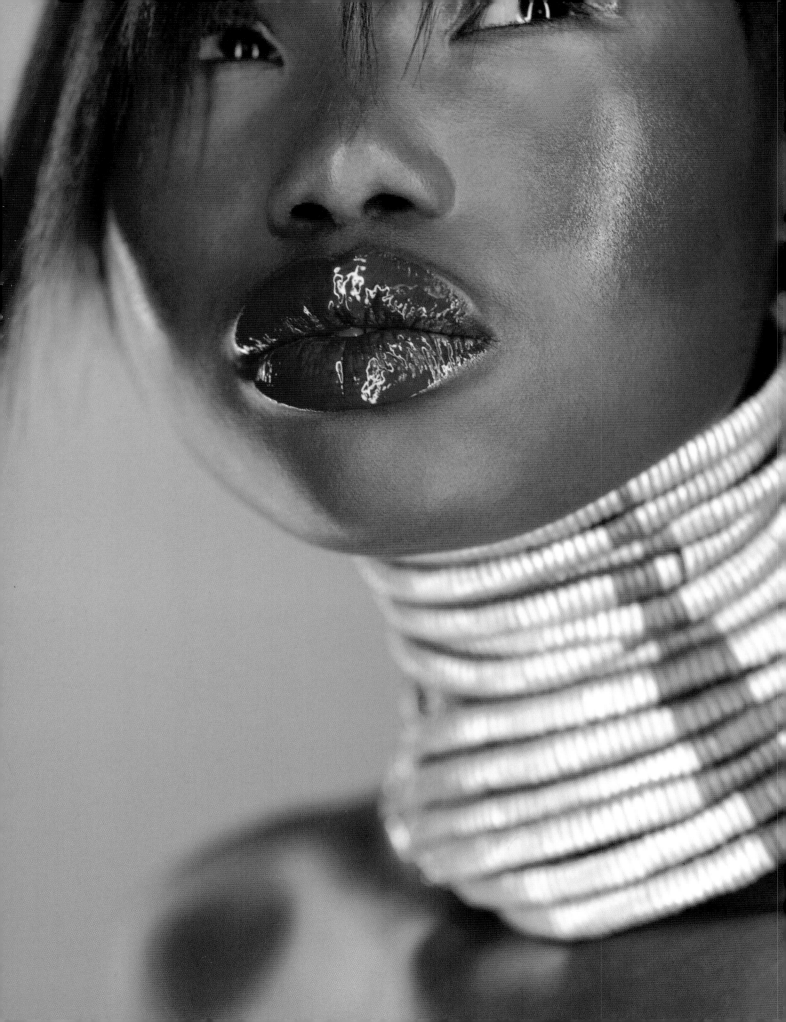

Who can do without blusher? The hard part is choosing the right formulation – if you've used face powder, then apply a powder blush; over foundation, opt for a cream blush; and on bare, moisturized skin, try a gel blush.

The plethora of colours available makes choices difficult, but sticking to rosy pinks and peaches works for most women. These shades enhance natural skin tone and are fairly forgiving if you're not that adept with the blusher brush. Don't be put off by shades that look very bright in the container; just a touch applied across the apple of the cheeks will result in a subtle finish.

The point of blusher is to add colour to the face, not to reshape it! Today make-up is all about being true to yourself. So, when applying make-up, play up your best features to minimize your weaker ones!

CHEEKS

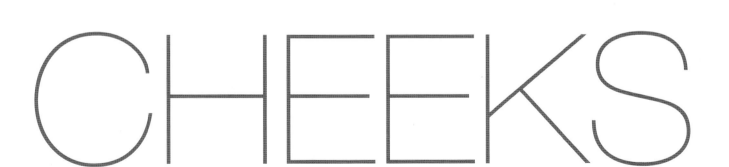

" Applied right, blusher gives a healthy flush. It energizes a tired face in seconds and creates wicked cheekbones. "

TEXTURE

These days blush comes in gels and creams. When applied well, it can play a number of roles. But whether the effect is evening glam or in-from-the-cold, it's essential that the colour looks a part of your skin, not sitting on top of it.

Powder blush. Easy to control and blend, and therefore the most popular choice, especially for oily skin. The downside is that you need a brush to apply powder, and it's hard to wipe off once you've put on too much. Once you have loaded a blusher brush with colour, tap off excess powder to avoid a harsh and unnatural look. Then work blusher from the centre of your cheeks out to the edges, working the brush in circular movements to blend.

Cream blush. New formulations spread easily. Good for dry and sun-damaged skin, sliding easily over the surface and not settling in wrinkles. Avoid if your skin is oily. Apply straight to your face and build up colour gradually. Ideally a cream blusher should be applied to unpowdered skin. Blend colour downward and outward to avoid demarcation lines.

Gel blush. Offers the sheerest form of colour, and is great for giving a natural-looking glow to bare skin. Great for applying to just-moisturized or nude skin. Blend from the apples of your cheeks outwards to avoid too much colour intensity at the hairline. Gels are ideal for a youthful, glowing look and are the easiest to apply. Blend quickly and don't forget to wash your stained fingers.

Bronzing powder. Can be substituted for blush in summer. It's also great dusted around the hairline, on the nose and chin, as well as across the cheekbones, for giving you a truly healthy-looking tan.

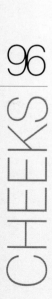

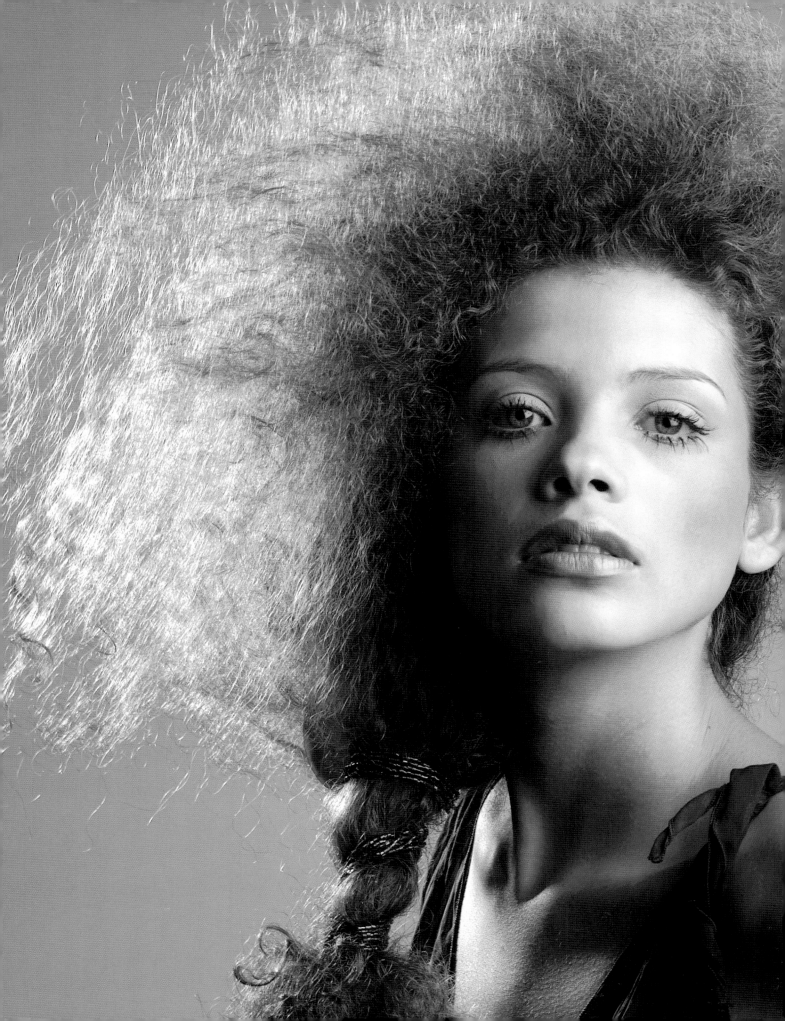

TRICKS
OF THE TRADE

- It's all about the right colour choice. If the blush is too obvious, you've got the wrong shade. Blush should add vitality and warmth to your complexion rather than alter your natural skin tone. Look for a shade that matches your skin when you blush naturally, usually pink or rosy tones. Test it on the back of your hand or, ideally, your cheeks, and examine the effect in natural daylight.

- Fair skins should stick to soft pastel shades with no brown in them: pale pinks. Medium skins work best with sandy, pink tones: peach and coral for redheads. Olive or yellow skins work best with pinky-rose colour. Avoid peach and bronze and look for brown and copper tones. Dark or black skins work best with rich shades of plum, fuchsia, deep bronze or burgundy.

- If you have broken veins or high colour, avoid blusher that has any red in it. Look for tawny or honey-coloured shades.

- What looks fabulous on catwalk models doesn't always translate into everyday wear. Bright fuchsia doll-like cheeks teamed with white highlighter are probably best suited to glossy magazine shoots or special occasions. Stick to gentler shades of pink or peach for a natural effect. Besides, they're much easier to apply.

- Emergency blush: blend a little lipstick into your cheeks for a creamy blush effect.

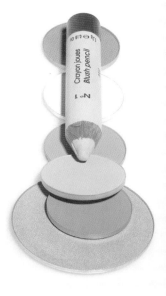

Common mistakes

■ Blush that is too shimmery can leave you looking ashen and grey.

■ Using shades that are too bright, dark or pale; blusher should never be noticeable.

■ Not blending enough can result in a horizontal stripe across cheeks.

■ Muddy or grey tones can leave skin looking dirty.

■ Blue and purple tones can make the skin look bruised.

■ Too much colour on the face; tap off excess before application or sweep translucent powder over the cheeks.

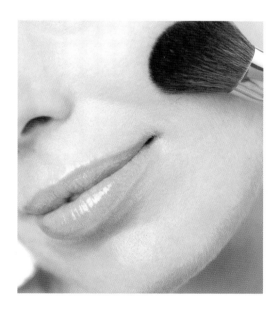

Anti-ageing

Our natural colouring fades as we age: lip colour becomes less pronounced, skin tone becomes less vibrant. If your colour is too pastel and discreet, you'll look washed out. So the trick is to carefully apply and blend more vibrant blush and lipstick colours.

Ultimately, blusher is the most effective make-up product for older skins. It can restore youth to a fading complexion, soften lines, blur sags and give skin a youthful glow. It can instantly take years off you by making you look healthier.

But where you wear your blusher today might not be where you wore it 10 years ago. Natural changes in the shape of the face demand a shift in make-up application techniques. Until we're about 35, we can wear blusher high on our cheekbones. When we start showing the first signs of age, we lose fatty tissue and form natural hollows under the cheekbones. At this point it becomes more flattering to use blusher towards the centre of the face and on the apples of the cheeks for a softer look.

Cream or gel-textured cheek colour is much more flattering for drier or post-30 skin. Why? It creates a soft, sheer, dewy finish and won't settle into fine lines and wrinkles like powder blush. Using the pad of your finger, dab a tiny dot of cream or gel onto the apples of your cheekbones, patting and blending until you're left with a natural, healthy glow.

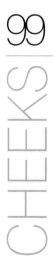

BLUSHER APPLICATION

1 **Find the apples of your cheeks.** Use this tried-and-tested technique: simply smile. Blush looks best when applied right on top of the cheekbones, which are right underneath the apples. Feel free to exaggerate your smile because putting colour too low can make you look as if you are trying to contour your cheek-bones, and putting it too close to the nose can make your face look heavy and narrow. The cheekbones also serve as a guide to keeping blush symmetrical.

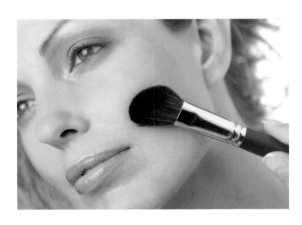

2 **Apply to cheeks.** With a brush, from which you've tapped the excess, or with a finger for a cream or gel, apply colour, starting at the point on your cheek directly below the middle of your eye. If you mis-takenly apply too much blush, wipe the excess off with a tissue before you blend.

3 **Blend the blush.** Swirl the colour onto your cheeks in circular, outward motions and blend upward towards your temple, keeping it fuller in the cheek area. Spend a little time brushing or rubbing the edges of the colour, until it flows smoothly into your natural skin colour. Make sure you use upward strokes to avoid disrupting the tiny facial hairs; they need to lie naturally.

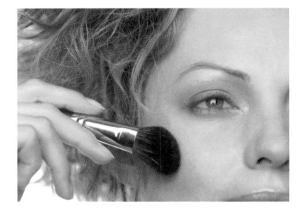

4 **A sun-kissed effect.** Apply blush or bronzer to the forehead, jawline, temples, chin, and the line down the centre of your nose – literally everywhere the sun would first touch your face. All-over blush works best in warm or bronze tones that are just a shade or two darker than your complexion. Put on as little as possible to avoid looking streaky or orange. Be more selective about where you place pink shades – they're not meant to go all over.

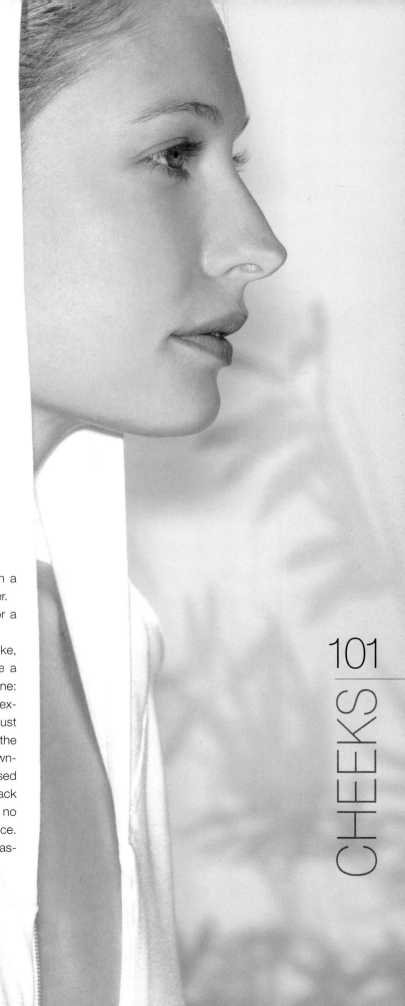

High cheekbones

▦ The most natural way to fake high cheekbones is with a cream or gel blush, which is easier to blend than powder.

▦ Find the apples of your cheeks and with your fingers or a sponge, work the blush outward in a circular motion.

▦ If your cheek bones aren't catching the light as you'd like, then a little highlighter will bring them forward. Choose a highlighter or shimmer stick to complement your skin tone: pale gold for fair skin or deep bronze for darker complexions. It doesn't have to be luminescent or shimmery, it just needs to be paler than the area you're highlighting. Dot the highlighter just above the cheekbones and blend downwards for a natural appearance, which takes a practised hand. This said, highlighting is useful for brightening black skins, provided you're using a highlighter that contains no titanium dioxide, which gives the skin an ashen appearance.

▦ Keep the rest of your make-up simple. Black or brown mascara and sheer gloss on the lips is all you need.

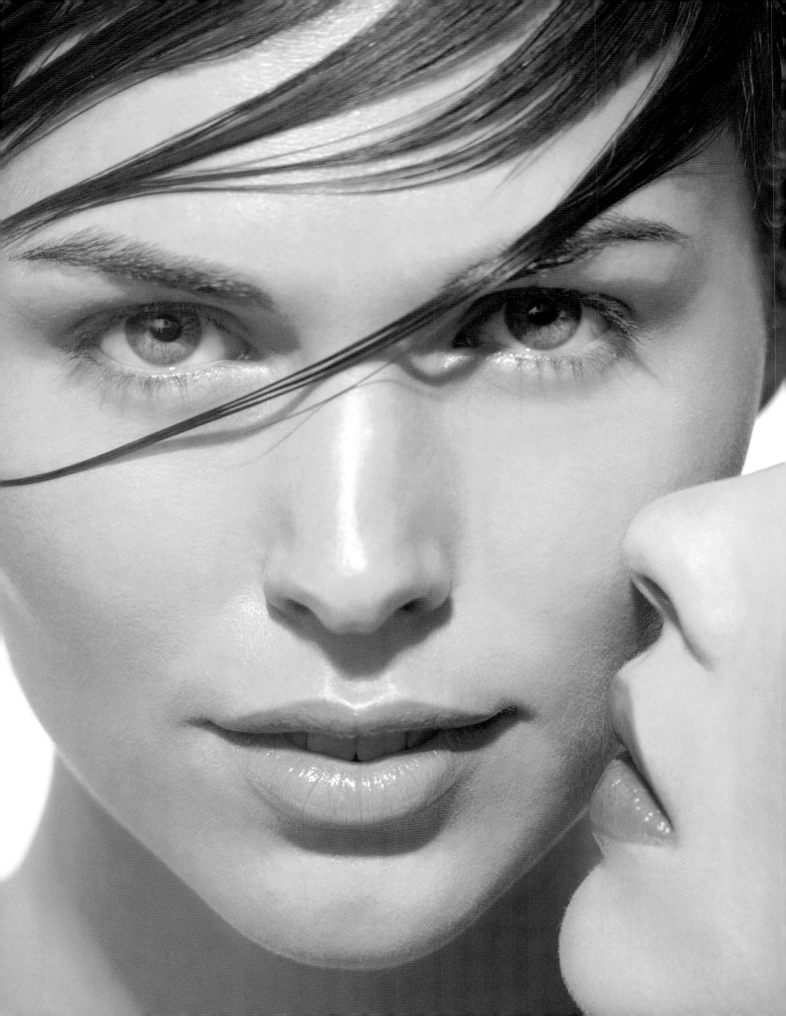

Make-up affords you unlimited possibilities – it allows you to be diva one minute and girl-next-door the next. You don't have to take beauty magazines literally – they're there to inspire you, to get you experimenting so that you can reinvent yourself.

Try to find a make-up style that makes you look and feel beautiful. Choose colours that will enhance your appearance and make-up techniques that look smooth and natural.

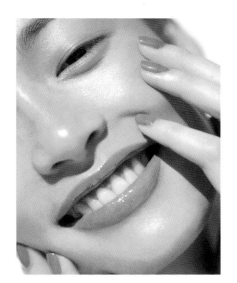

LOOKS

"Trends are meant to innovate and inspire and should not be taken too literally ..."

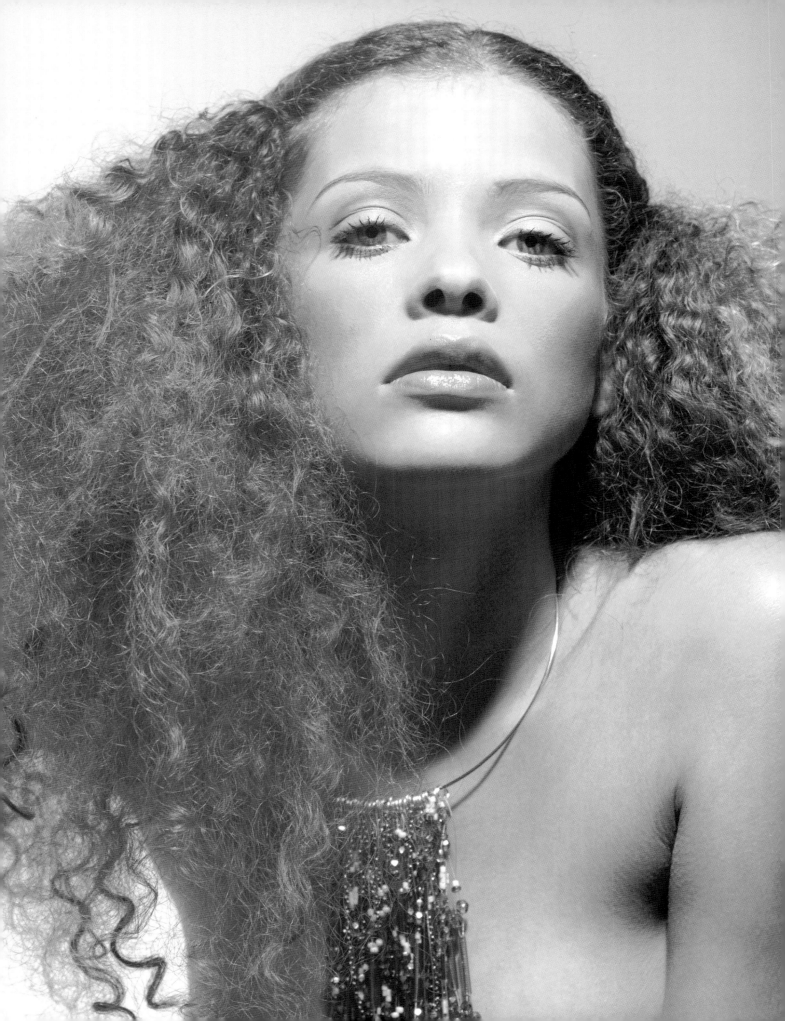

BASIC MAKE-UP

This look is easy to achieve and can be worked with any set of colours,
but the brown and beige tones we've used are neutral shades that will never go out of style.
They're earthy and soft, easy to blend and go with just about anything.
You can simply intensify the tone to get a more dramatic look or play up one aspect
like we did with the eyelashes to create impact.

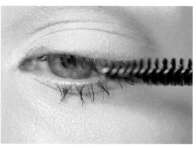

Pick a light, a dark, and a medium shade of shadow. It's easier when they belong to the same colour family, but not essential. The trick is remembering what each tone is supposed to do.

The lightest shade opens up the eye area – dust onto the entire lid, from brow to lash line. The medium shade contours the crease line. The darkest shade adds emphasis to the eyes – apply with small angled brush to outer corners of eyes close to the lash line.

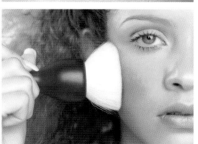

We left out the darkest shade and focused on the lashes instead, applying one coat of mascara and powdering the lashes before applying the next coat for a thicker, spikier Seventies look.

Contour cheeks. Set foundation with a very light dusting of powder and contour cheek hollows with a sweep of natural blush using a big blusher or blending brush. Blend colour carefully.

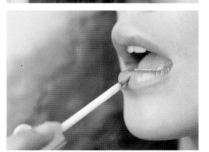

Use a gloss wand on the centre of the lips, then blend up and out to the lip line. When applying gloss straight from the tube, start from the middle of the mouth and work towards the corners.

Tips
- Most neutral shades blend easily; the lighter the application, the more natural the look. Intensify the tone for a more dramatic evening look.
- A neutral blusher shade won't sculpt your cheek bones as much as it will give you a healthy glow.

SUN KISSED

No matter how often we're told never to bake our faces in the sun, many still believe that there's no summer accessory as beautiful as warm glowing skin. Ultimately, a radiant, bronzed face is still the hottest beauty trend around ... so fake it!

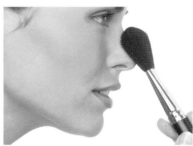

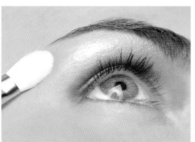

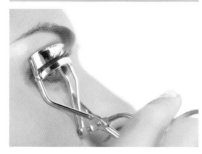

Switch to a tinted moisturizer in the heat. It offers UV protection and a fresh, radiant glow. Change to a stick foundation if you feel the need to even out skin tone, cover blemishes or disguise dark circles.

Blusher isn't essential, but a touch of bronzing cream or powder high on the cheekbones creates a subtle glow that makes you look sun kissed days before you are. Apply bronzing powder with a short, fluffy brush wherever the sun would hit naturally – forehead, cheekbones, bridge of nose, and your neck. If you have smooth, dry skin, try using bronzing sticks or creams in a sheer formulation and apply with your fingers or a sponge.

Make lashes the focus, forget shadows and eye-pencils. If you want to wear make-up on top of your tan, choose shades that add light to your face and help prevent it from looking too flat. A touch of iridescent or golden colour works on the centre of the eyelid, below the brows and in the inner corners of the eyes.

An eyelash curler is an indispensable aid for maximizing your lashes. To curl your lashes, look straight into the mirror, position the curler carefully over the lashes, at their base, before pressing firmly down on the curler for five to ten seconds. Roll curler slightly up and away while holding the grip, then repeat for the other eye. Always curl lashes before applying mascara, or you might damage your lashes.

Tips

- On the beach, apply sunscreen to face and body first thing.
- Bronzing powder can double up over foundation as eye shadow and blusher. If last year's bronzing powder now looks too ginger, dip your brush into loose translucent powder first to dilute it.
- A tan is sheer, not opaque, so simply using a darker shade of foundation won't work.
- Dry skin and fake tan don't work together. Exfoliate regularly for healthier-looking results.
- To cope with holiday heat and humidity, switch to an oil-free foundation or tinted moisturizer.

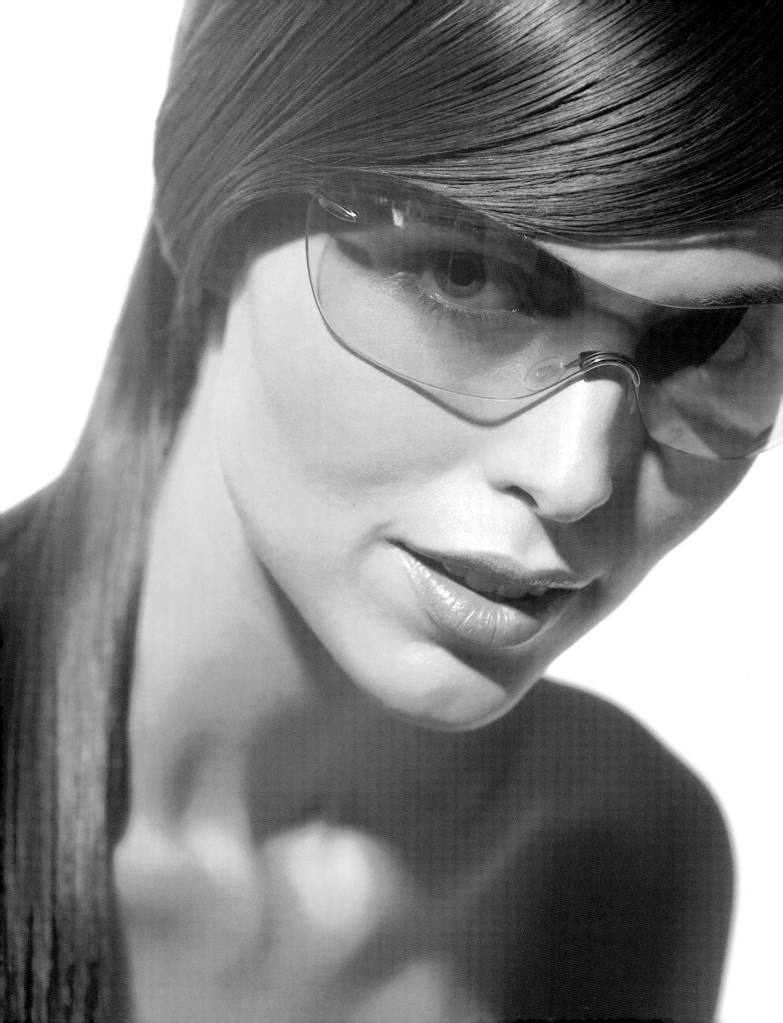

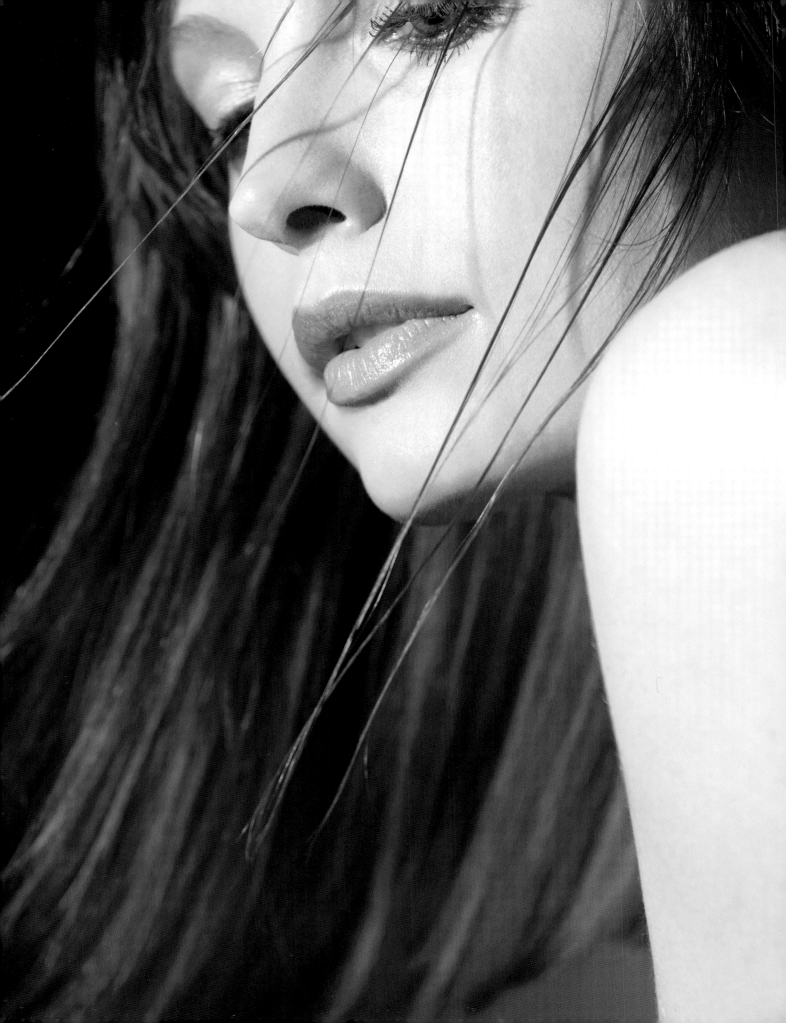

The natural or 'barely there' look is probably one of the hardest to achieve, as it needs a light, skilful touch and careful choice of colour. Natural means enhancing your natural look with as little make-up as possible. Use little to no foundation, especially in summer when your skin has more colour. Warm, earthy, neutral tones work best – anything from pale vanilla and almond to mid-tones like taupe and terracotta to deeper shades like coffee and brown. Colour choice is personal, although redheads look great in brick-browns and brunettes look stunning in mocha!

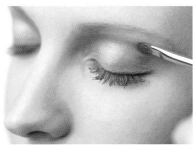

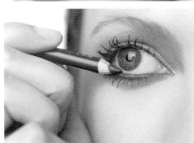

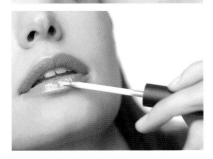

Moisturize and apply a convincing shade of liquid foundation if necessary. Conceal problem areas, making sure you blend carefully. Set concealer and foundation with loose powder, using a velour puff. Dust the apples of your cheeks with a soft shade of blusher to create a healthy glow.

Use a shadow brush to apply the lightest shade of eye shadow all over the lid, from the lash line to the eyebrow. Then brush a medium shade of shadow across the entire lid, from the lashes to just above the crease line, and blend. Apply the darkest shade along the lash line as close to the lashes as possible, placing added emphasis on the outer corners.

Line eyes inside the inner rim and around the outer edges with a soft, brown kajal eye pencil. Apply one or two coats of mascara. Brush eyebrows into shape and define if necessary with eye shadow.

Define lips with a neutral shade of lipliner pencil and fill with lipstick. If you wish, slick with gloss, but remember that leaving it off will make your lipstick last longer.

Tip

■ Careful blending is essential. The aim is to give the complexion a healthy glow by using foundation and blusher that subtly enhance your natural skin tone rather than disguise it.

SMOKY

No matter how dramatic, a smoky eye will always be soft and velvety. This is a glamorous high-maintenance look and the key is careful blending with darker colours – grey, brown, purple, deep green, charcoal, navy ... Let the darkest shade at the lash line grow gradually lighter as you move away from it; create the impression that you've used one colour.

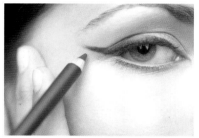

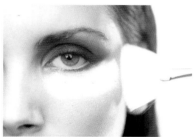

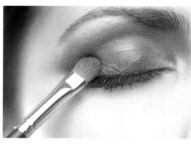

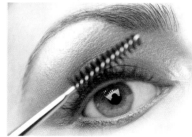

Spread a little concealer onto the upper and lower lids to cover veins and prevent creasing. Curl your lashes and apply eyeliner according to your eye shape: if you have close-set eyes, apply pencil liner only to the outer corner, otherwise line the entire upper lid. Pull the eyelid gently at the outer corner, so that the eyeliner glides on smoothly in an even line. To make eyes look longer, extend the eyeliner beyond the outer corners.

Powder liberally under the eyes to prevent spill-off, then brush powder eye shadow in the same shade as the liner over the lines to soften them and keep the liner from rubbing off. Apply the same shade along the lower lid, close underneath the lashes.

Brush a highlighter across the browbone to dramatize the eye area. Blend carefully and clean up mistakes or smudges with a cotton bud. Apply two light coats of mascara to the upper and lower lashes, combing through to separate and declog.

Outline lips with a lip pencil that matches your lipstick, then fill the entire area with lipstick using a lip brush to get into the corners.

Tips

- Keep eyeliner pencils sharpened, but soften by drawing a line on your hand before applying to sensitive areas.
- As a beginner, start with pencil liner, which is easier to control and offers a softer look. If you can't draw a straight line, draw connected dashes along your lash line. Ensure that no skin shows between eyelid and lash roots.
- Use an eye shadow or kohl pencil along the bottom inner rim of the eye, taking it right into the corner.

LOOKS

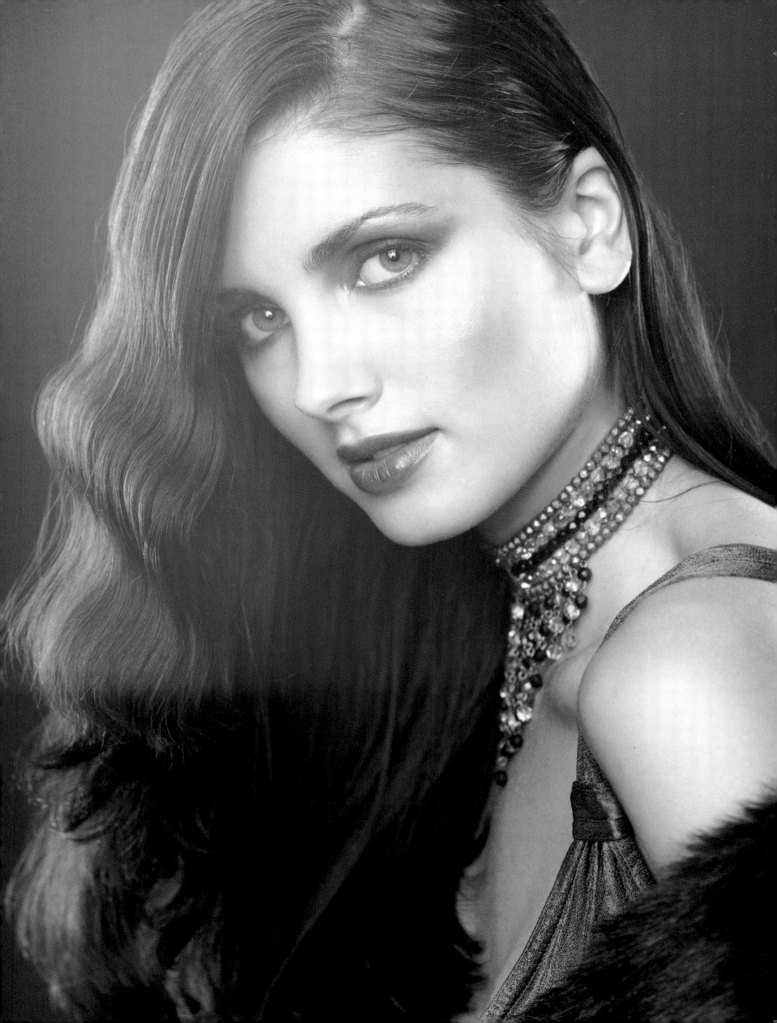

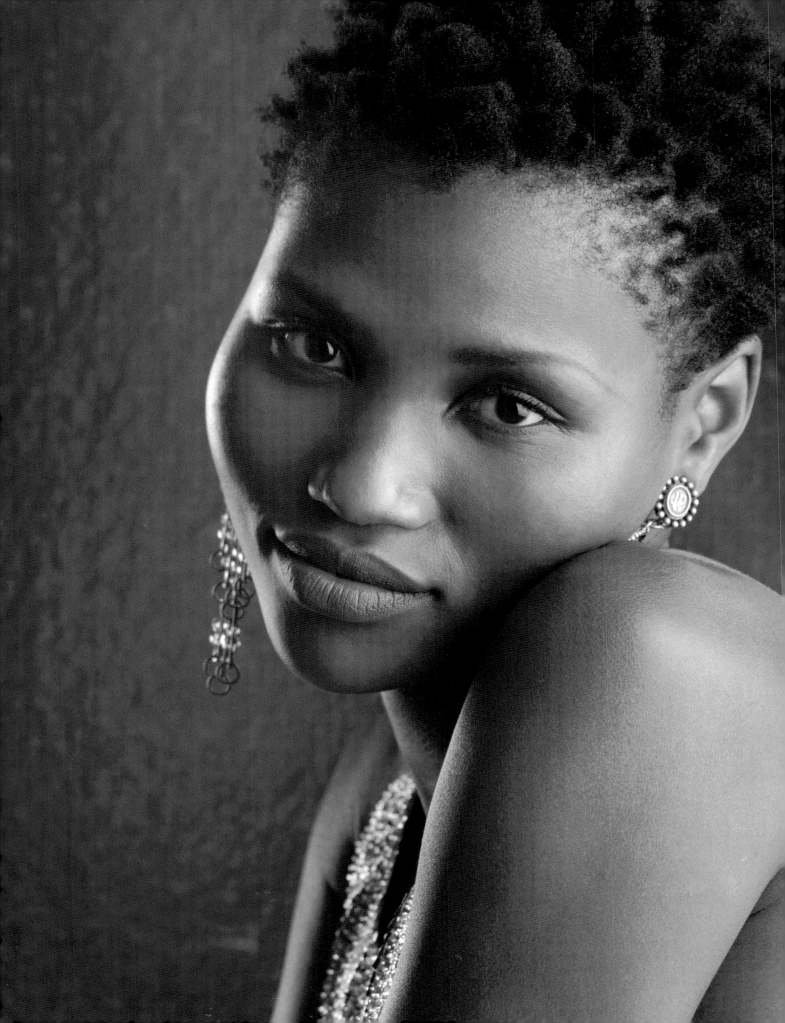

The biggest problem for black skins is finding the right shade of foundation, but most cosmetic companies have addressed this problem and are constantly adding new, darker shades to their ranges. Shadow and powder colours devised for darker skins usually contain deeper pigment levels, which ensure true colour on the skin. Many black women are darker across the forehead and chin, and lighter on the cheekbones. Even this out by applying a lighter shade of foundation on the forehead and chin areas and a slightly darker shade on the cheek area.

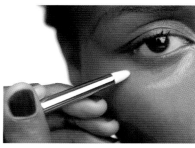

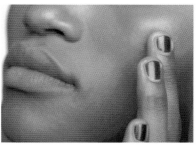

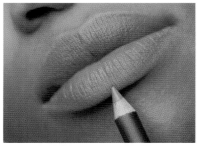

Prep your skin with an oil-free moisturizer, then use a concealer one or two tones lighter than your skin tone to correct under-eye shadows and blemishes.

Using a damp sponge, dot foundation onto the forehead, cheeks, nose and chin and begin blending outward and downward. Set with a light dusting of powder.

Prime the eyelid area with a dusting of translucent powder. Smudge the darker tone of eye shadow around the outer corners of the eyes and along the crease line to create depth.

Use the lighter shade on the inner corners. If eyebrows need added definition, use an eyebrow brush and pencil. Blend and apply lots of mascara.

Use a lip brush to fill in lips and correct the lip line. To give a richer colour to the lipstick and increase staying power, apply lip pencil to the entire lip area.

Tips
- Berry-coloured lip gloss blended onto the cheeks gives a moist, glowing look.
- Apply foundation first to balance lip colour and make lipstick last longer.
- Avoid foundations with SPF that contains zinc dioxide.

SHIMMER EYES

Iridescent or metallic eye make-up is a great accessory to dewy or light-reflecting foundations. This look is about choosing whatever colour you fancy and using it in a soft and pretty way. There are no hard edges – only soft, subtle, blended colour. Use intense colour only on your eyes, with neutral cheeks and lips for maximum impact, or try using intense colour only on your lips and keep the rest of your make-up pale. Play up one feature for a truly modern feel.

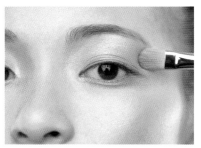

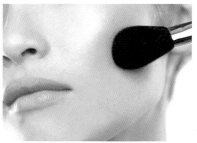

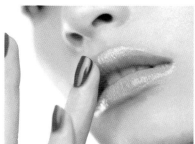

Apply a sweep of green eye shadow to the top lid and extend upward at the outer corner and slightly under the eye. Choose another, darker shade of eye shadow and sweep underneath the eye, blending outwards. Blend under the eyes with a cotton bud. Blend the lightest shade into the inner corner on the top lid. Work the colour out to the crease to diffuse and soften the green shade.

Finish eyes with black mascara. Use a cotton bud to blend any fall-out under the eyes for a dramatic look. Brush eyebrows into shape and seal with a clear mascara or try squirting some hairspray onto an old toothbrush and brush it through the brows for a lasting hold.

Blend a rosy shade of blusher on the cheekbones, working under the cheekbone outline to create a contour effect.

On the lips fingertip application is easier – less tidy but also less defined than lip brush application. Use two shades of lipstick – the lighter shade is added to the centre of the top and bottom lips as a highlight.

LOOKS

Tips
- Blend colours carefully so you can't discern where one shade starts and the other ends.
- Add depth by applying the darker colour slightly above the crease line.

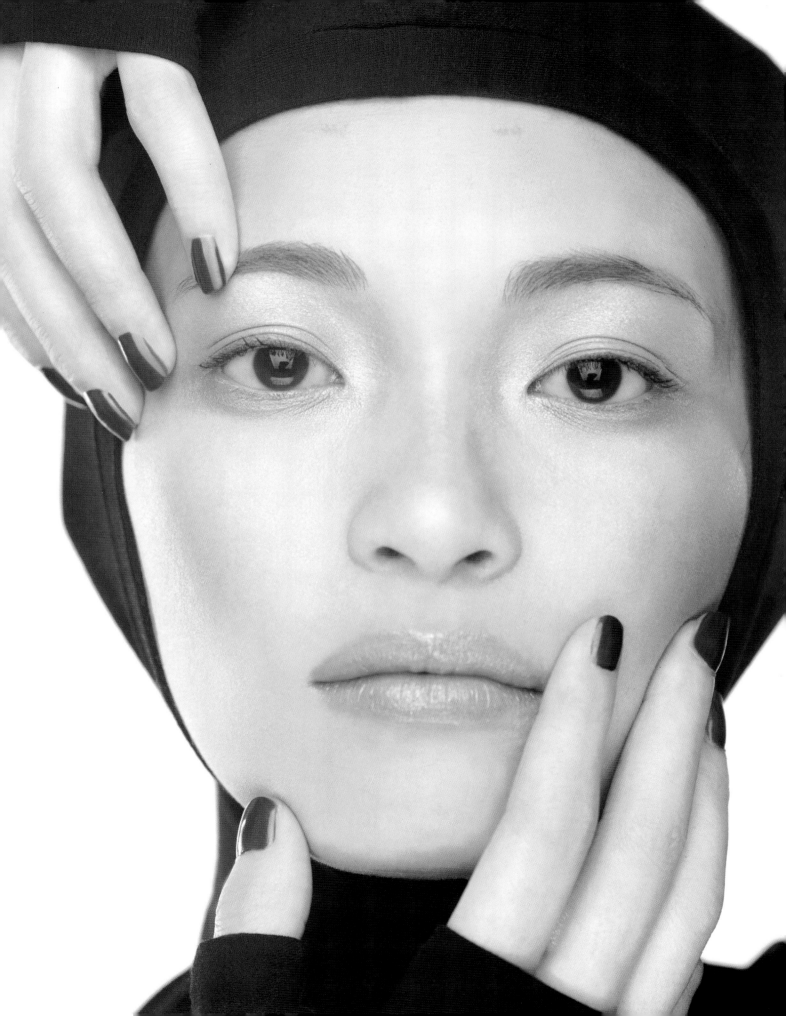

TEENAGE

Make-up for teenagers should enhance rather than conceal. This is a time for experimentation, when texture, colour, shimmer won't detract from your single biggest asset – your youth! Keep your make-up simple and natural and look for products that you can apply with your fingertips. Transparent, pale and pastel colours are easy to apply and pretty mistake-proof too.

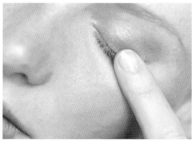

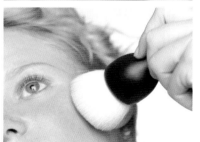

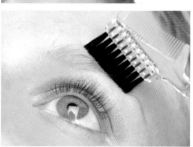

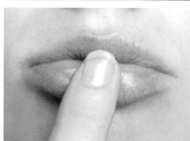

Apply foundation to cover any unevenness if necessary. Take care to blend in carefully. Use a powder puff to pat a little powder over your face to set foundation, shaking off excess before you start.

Sweep a shimmery eye shadow across the eyelid and blend with fingertips or a sponge-tipped applicator.

Swirl the blusher colour onto your cheeks in a circular outward motion or simply dot cream blusher onto cheeks. Start at the point on your cheek directly below the middle of your eye and blend with fingertips to create a natural flush.

Mascara goes onto the top and bottom lashes with extra emphasis on outer and top lashes. Brush eyebrows up slightly and then along, to neaten any spiky hairs.

Prime your lips with a good cream, then rub them with a soft toothbrush to get rid of any dead or dry skin cells. Apply lip colour with fingertips; press lips together to work in the pigment. High shine will make your lips the focal point of your face, but remember anything too glossy will need constant retouching.

Tips
- Avoid using a magnifying mirror – it will only depress you!
- Stay away from heavy foundations – they're definitely out.
- Experiment, make mistakes – you can always wash them off.

LOOKS

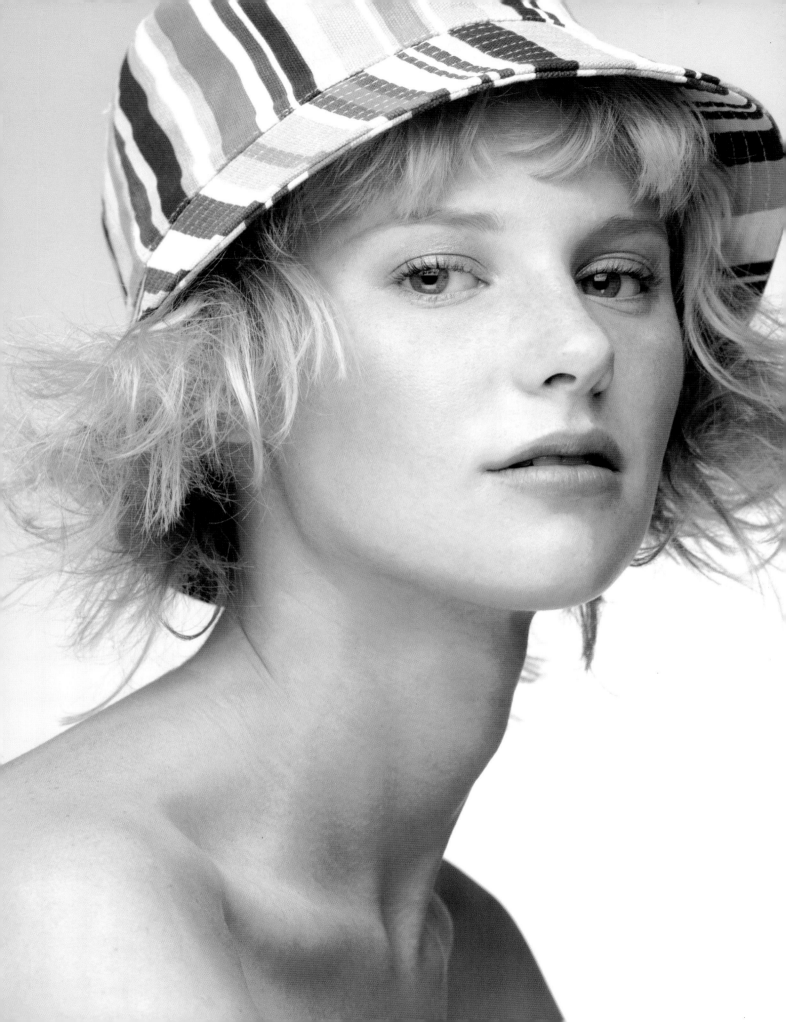

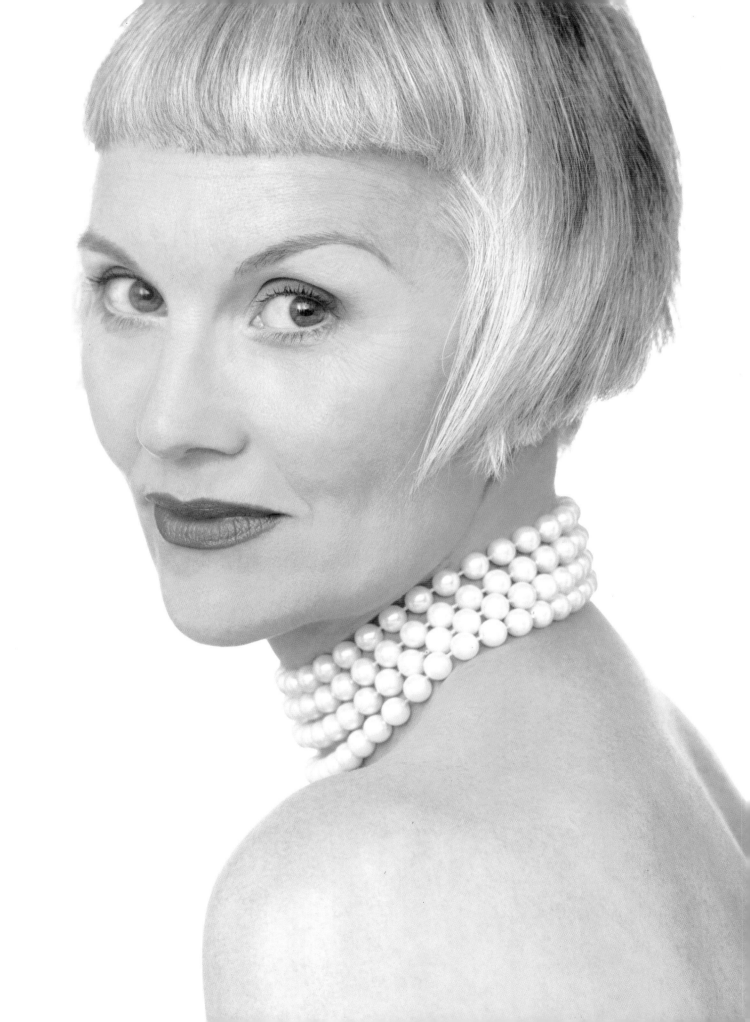

MATURE

Our natural colouring fades as we age – lip colour becomes less pronounced and skin tone becomes less vibrant. Blusher and lipstick can restore youth to a fading complexion, soften lines and provide a youthful glow. However, as we mature, we also need to change our application techniques. After about 35, we lose fatty tissue and form natural hollows. So it becomes more flattering to place blusher towards the centre of the face and on the apples of the cheeks.

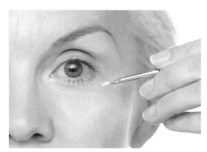

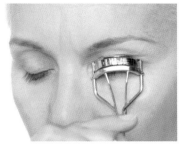

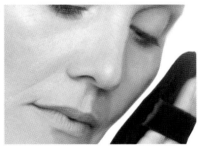

Moisturize and apply a light-reflecting foundation that makes lines and skin tone less noticeable. Apply a light-reflecting concealer with a fine brush to minimize blemishes, shadows and pigmentation marks. Set make-up with a light dusting of powder, but not too much or it'll settle into fine lines. Powder can be very ageing if applied incorrectly. Use a velour sponge to roll and blot powder to avoid overdoing it.

Emphasize the eyelashes to give definition to the face, especially if your lashes have lost their colour. Use eyelash curlers before applying mascara. Holding them below the eye, place the curlers so that the upper lashes are in the gap between the two rims, then squeeze for a few seconds before removing. Finally apply mascara to the upper lashes from below and to the lower lashes from above, using less mascara on the lower lashes.

Let blusher restore a youthful glow to a fading complexion – just think pink. Powder blush can look very harsh on mature skins; instead choose a cream blusher, which glides on easily.

Stick to warm pinkish tones for the lips and use a lip pencil the same colour as your lips to outline and fill your mouth – the waxy texture of the lip pencil will prevent the lipstick from 'bleeding' or 'feathering' into fine lines.

Tips
- Avoid matte foundation formulations, which emphasize dull skin.
- Apply less foundation around the far edges of the eyes, where it may draw attention to fine lines.
- Avoid liquid eyeliner. Try pencil or powder shadow applied with a blunt brush instead.
- Avoid frosted iridescent shadows containing mica, a pearlized powder that settles in wrinkles.

SPEED

This is one of the easiest and quickest looks to achieve. Provided your skin is generally clear, skip foundation and concealer and simply use a tinted moisturizer if you need a touch of colour. If your skin isn't clear, look for stick foundations, or simply use the concealer where you need it and powder to set. Creamy eye shadow and lipstick formulations that you can apply with your fingertips also help speed the process, allowing you to do your make-up on the run.

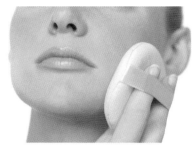

Dab a creamy concealer wherever you need it: around your nose, at the corners of your mouth, on under-eye circles and at the outer corners of your eyes. Apply a light foundation, blending it quickly down the T-panel and chin areas or dabbing only onto the areas that need it. Set with a very light dusting of powder.

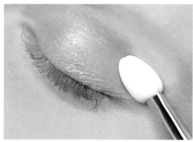

Blend a creamy eye shadow over the entire eyelid, being careful not to go beyond the crease line. Use your fingertips or a sponge-tipped applicator to blend. Apply two coats of a curling or thickening mascara and use a mascara comb or brush to separate lashes. Brush eyebrows to remove any excess powder.

Sweep a natural gel or cream-based blusher colour onto the apples of your cheeks, using your fingertips. Build colour gradually, working the colour downward and outward to avoid an obvious cut-off line.

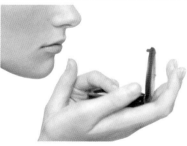

Skip lipliner and put on lipstick straight from the tube. Dab lipstick onto the centre of your lips and smear outwards with your fingertips. Press lips together to work in the pigment. Blot so just a stain of colour is left and cover generously with lip balm or gloss. Be prepared to reapply often – balm and gloss wear off quickly.

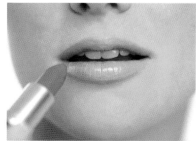

Tips

- Don't use anything too dark, or you'll spend too much time neatening and reapplying. Translucence is the order of the day.
- Look for creamy formulations of eye shadow that are easy to smudge and smear with your fingertips. Chubby sticks in creamy formulations are also a quick way out.

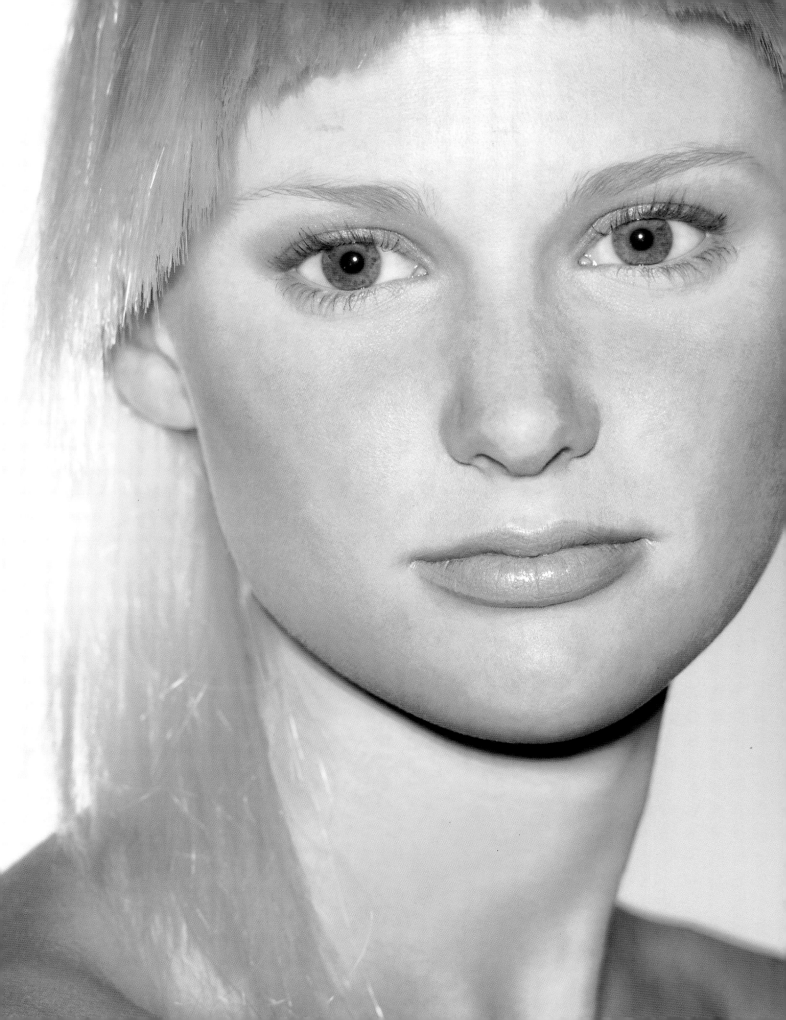

LOVE THAT CAMERA

The trick with photographic make-up is to get the skin tone right – a photographer's flash intensifies the pink in foundations and face powders, so yellow-toned products are more effective. You need good definition in your make-up if the photographer is using black-and-white film. Harsh, high-contrast studio lighting means that blush becomes very important. Usually flaws are softened and skin can look flat and lifeless if you're not using the right colours.

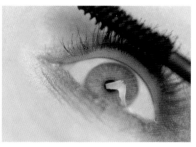

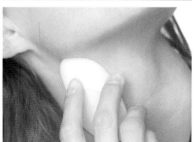

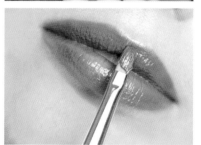

Apply matte eye shadow and blusher – shimmery products will only look greasy in the finished photograph – then two coats of mascara for extra definition. Allow each coat to dry thoroughly before applying the next. Comb through to separate lashes.

Carefully blend foundation into neckline and shoulders. One of the biggest problems about make-up in photographs is the face looking whiter than the rest of the body – so match your foundation to the skin tone of your chest and neck, rather than your face, to eliminate this problem. Pay particular attention to demarcation lines along the jaw line; blend thoroughly.

Avoid brown or beige lip tones. For a finished look apply lipliner using a lip brush for added definition. Highlight the cupid's bow (the centre of the upper lip) using either a lip gloss or a paler shade of lipstick, then highlight the centre of the bottom lip to create the illusion of fullness.

Tips

- Blend foundation down your neck and chest for effective cover and an even skin tone, but bear in mind that it will rub off onto your clothes, so only do this for pictures.
- Warm tones of powder and foundation help prevent that washed-out look.
- Blush is critical for the definition of the face.

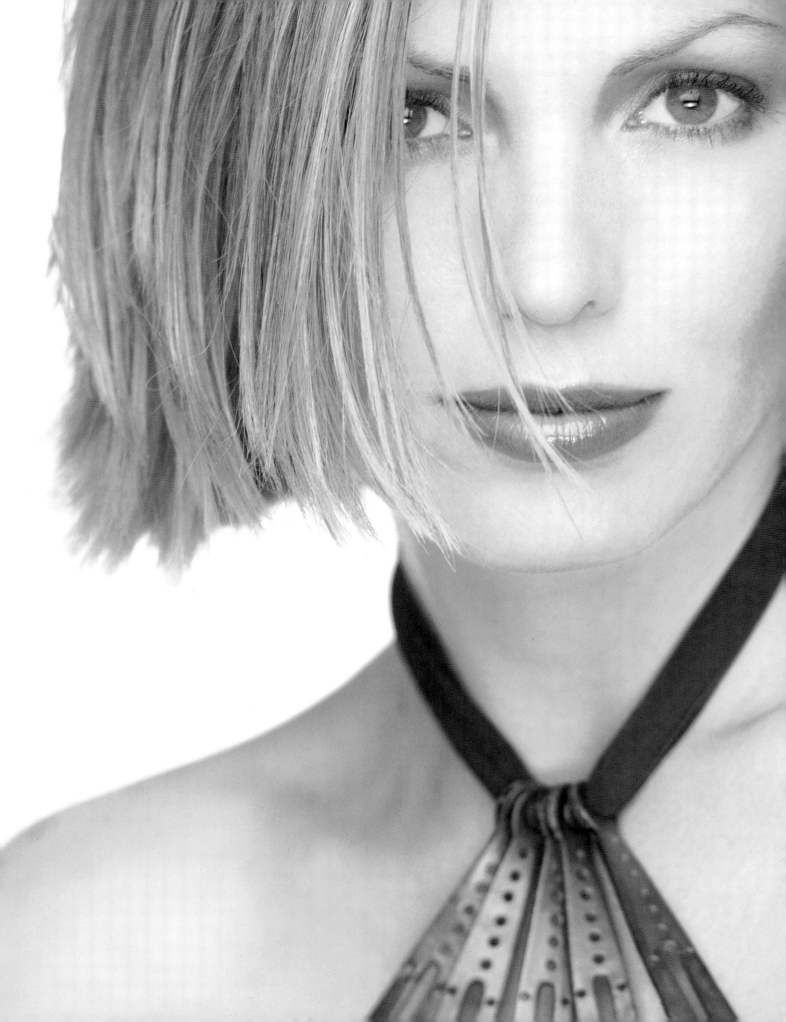

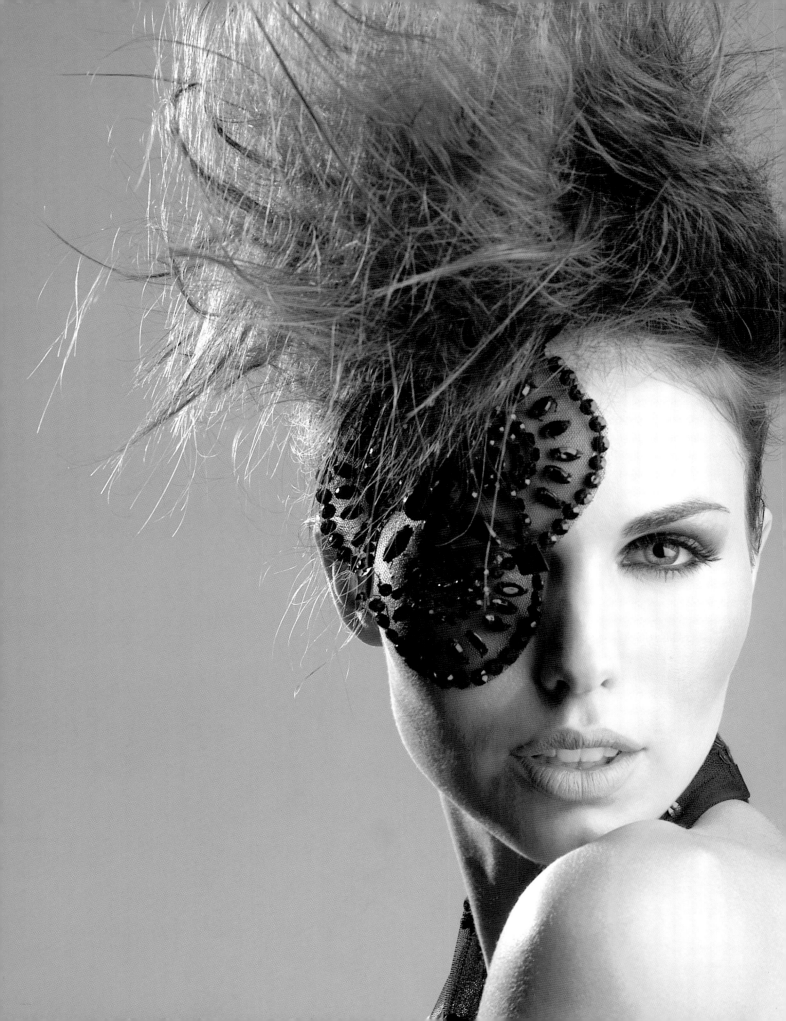

GLAM

Distinctive dark, dramatic eyes and pale-coloured lips are not for the faint-hearted. This dramatic evening look can be softened by a delicate shade of lipstick. Charcoal shadow practically encircles the eyes, while the top and bottom lashes are lined for emphasis with eyeliner and false lashes. False eyelashes aren't for everyone, but a practised hand can add drama by enhancing and lengthening your top lashes – they aren't as difficult to put on as you might think.

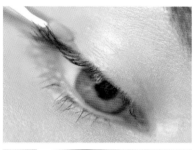

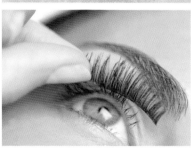

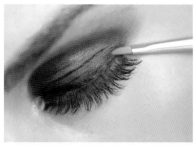

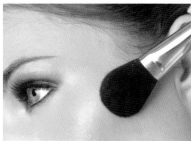

Holding the skin slightly taut, position your eye pencil at the inner corner of your eye, resting on top of your lashes. Sweep the upper lash line to the outer corner, drawing outward. Brush over with a small, pointed eye shadow brush to softly smudge the pencil.

Pick up the false eyelash using a pair of tweezers and run a small amount of glue along the top edge; wait a few seconds for the glue to dry slightly. Line up the outer edge of the false lash against the outer edge of your own lash, and then gently push as close as possible into the roots. Make sure the eyelash is properly secure at the outer and inner corners. Keep your eye closed for a little while as the glue dries, then run a thin line of liquid eyeliner over the join to give a neat finish. Finally line the bottom lid with a pencil line.

Apply a grey eye shadow on the lid. Work this colour up past the crease. For added impact apply a little Vaseline over the shadow. This technique is very trendy right now but can make the eye shadow slip and slide. If you want an effect that will last, leave out this step.

Finish the face with a bit of rosy shimmer on the cheekbones and a subtle pale pink lipstick.

Tips
- By curling your eyelashes before you apply the false ones, you create a better contour for the lashes to sit against.
- Play up one feature – we focused on the eyes and under-played the mouth for a contemporary feel.

LOOKS

GLOSSARY

From AHAs to retinol, the beauty business can blind you with science. Here are a few common terms:

Alpha-hydroxy acids (AHAs) Also known as fruit acids and derived from natural substances such as milk, wine and apples, AHAs brighten the complexion by loosening flaky, dead skin cells and encouraging natural cell turnover. AHAs may cause mild irritation and slight tingling to sensitive skin.

Antioxidants These are substances found in plants, vitamins and food that protect against cell-destroying free radicals. Some claim they have a dramatic effect on wrinkles; others believe levels of antioxidant vitamins C, E and betacarotene in creams are too low to be effective. Natural antioxidants in beauty products include green algae, grape seed extract, rosemary and liquorice. Ginkgo biloba and green tea are known to be the strongest.

Ascorbic acid This is a water-based form of vitamin C that is commonly found in anti-ageing creams. It is known to help diminish fine lines and increase 'plumpness' by stimulating the production of collagen and elastin, proteins essential for a healthy complexion. It is also used as a cosmetic preservative.

Ceramides These are lipids or fats found between the cells of the outer layer of the skin (the stratum corneum), which help your skin retain moisture. Many products designed for older, dry sun-damaged and dehydrated skin types contain ceramides.

Collagen A key element of the skin's support structure, collagen keeps it smooth, supple and youthful, but breaks down with age, causing the skin to sag. It is usually derived either from cows or from human donations after breast reduction operations. It is used in injections to plump out wrinkles and is also found in many skin creams, although these cannot 'fill' the skin in the same way as an injection can and are generally more useful for their moisturizing qualities.

Comedogenic A term used to describe an ingredient that tends to create a blockage of the follicle and cause the formation of blackheads.

Cosmoceutical A combination of the terms cosmetic and pharmaceutical. This term is becoming increasingly popular to describe cosmetic preparations with biological claims. Some describe them as cosmetic drugs that include anti-ageing creams, anti-wrinkle lotions, and similar products.

Free radicals These are molecules that damage normal cells by depleting them of oxygen. Our bodies create them when exposed to sunlight, pollution or stress. They can lead to cell breakdown, resulting in premature ageing or diseases such as cancer. Antioxidants can help fight against free radicals.

Humectant This is the generic name for ingredients, such as glycerine, that attract moisture from the atmosphere to the surface of the skin, thus increasing the skin's moisture content. Humectants have the ability to bind moisture and are considered moisturizers.

Hypoallergenic A cosmetic product that does not produce allergic reactions. Usually this term is applied to products that are fragrance free and that have a select type of preservative. However products containing essential oils and plant extracts pose a greater risk of allergic reactions.

Liposomes These are microscopic bubbles that carry other substances and help deliver moisture to the skin. They were originally developed by doctors to target a drug to a specific area of the body. The idea was taken up by the skin-care industry more than a decade ago to carry nourishing ingredients into the skin to 'plump it up' and reduce the appearance of fine lines. However, products containing liposomes still only penetrate the top layer of the skin – if they penetrated further, they would be classified as drugs rather than as cosmetics.

Lymphatic system This is the body's 'drainage network', where harmful toxins are filtered from the circulation by the lymph nodes, to protect against infection.

Melanin This is the colour pigment responsible for your natural skin tone. In addition, melanin is the body's natural sun-defence mechanism: during exposure to UV (ultraviolet) rays, the body produces melanin to protect the skin, giving you a tan in the process.

pH balance This measures the acidity or alkalinity of the skin, and is graded on a scale of 1 to 14. A pH7 is neutral; below 7 is acidic and above 7 is alkaline. The natural pH balance of the skin is between 5 and 6.

Pigmentation There are two types: hypopigmentation, where patches of skin are paler because pigment is reduced, often due to ageing; and hyperpigmentation, often called liver spots, due to an excess of pigment.

INDEX

ACKNOWLEDGEMENTS

Photography: Patrick Toselli
Photographic assistant: Michael Linders
Make-up artists: Lesley Whitby, Michel Ingoglia and Melody Cokayne.
Hairdressers: Saadique Ryklief, Guilliame Nel and Karen Meadows
Models: Cecile, Kirsten, Andy, Ming Yong of Heads Model Agency; Naomi at Fork Models; Mary at Tribe Models; May at Icons; Edith and Ronwyn at Noir Models.
Stylist: Kim Berell

The author would also like to thank the following companies and individuals for their help in producing this book: Make-Up For Ever for the use of their products and Melissa Brown for her invaluable input; Clarins for the use of their skin-care products and Debbie Wolfendale's tireless knowledge; Clinique for their assistance and use of their products; MAC for the use of their make-up and brushes; Jackie Burger for allowing us to experiment with her face and for trusting the process; Migi for his endless cups of tea; stylist Kim Berell for finding such beautiful clothes and accessories; Saadique Ryklief, Guilliame Nel and Karen Meadows for their great hairdos; make-up artists Melody Cokayne, Lesley Whitby and Michel Ingoglia for their amazing attention to detail and passion for this project. Thanks for the perfectly 'painted' faces – your expertise has been invaluable over the years. Thanks also to the models – Cecile, Kirsten, Andy, Ming Yong, Naomi, Mary, May, Ronwyn and Edith – for your help, enthusiasm and versatility; Delyse Harding for reading and rereading the text and for getting me into this field in the first place (thanks, Mom!); Alfred LeMaitre for his patience; Petal Palmer for her beautiful design; Devin, Rowan and Kieran Toselli for their endless support, back-up and patience in waiting for me to finish yet another page of copy before helping with homework; and, last but not least, Patrick for his unerring eye and devotion to photographing beautiful women and, of course, our brilliant working relationship – together we are formidable!